Pharmaceuticals and Society

Sociology of Health and Illness Monograph Series

Edited by Hannah Bradby
Department of Sociology
University of Warwick
Coventry
CV4 7AL
UK

Current titles:

Pharmaceuticals and Society
Critical Discourses and Debates

Edited by

Simon J. Williams, Jonathan Gabe, and Peter Davis

WILEY-BLACKWELL

A John Wiley & Sons, Ltd., Publication

First published as volume 30, issue 6 of *Sociology of Health & Illness*

Blackwell Publishing was acquired by John Wiley & Sons in February 2007. Blackwell's publishing program has been merged with Wiley's global Scientific, Technical, and Medical business to form Wiley-Blackwell.

Registered Office
John Wiley & Sons Ltd, The Atrium, Southern Gate, Chichester, West Sussex, PO19 8SQ, United Kingdom

Editorial Offices
350 Main Street, Malden, MA 02148-5020, USA
9600 Garsington Road, Oxford, OX4 2DQ, UK
The Atrium, Southern Gate, Chichester, West Sussex, PO19 8SQ, UK

For details of our global editorial offices, for customer services, and for information about how to apply for permission to reuse the copyright material in this book please see our website at www.wiley.com/wiley-blackwell.

Library of Congress Cataloging-in-Publication Data

Pharmaceuticals and society : critical discourses and debates / edited by Simon J. Williams, Jonathan Gabe, and Peter Davis.
    p. cm. — (Sociology of health and illness monograph series)
    Includes bibliographical references and index.
    ISBN 978-1-4051-9084-8 (pbk. : alk. paper) 1. Drug abuse—Great Britain. 2. Drugs—Social aspects—Great Britain. 3. Drug abuse. 4. Drugs—Social aspects. I. Williams, Simon J. (Simon Johnson), 1961– II. Gabe, Jonathan. III. Davis, Peter.
    HV5840. P43 2009
    362.29'90941–dc22

                                       2008043813

A catalogue record for this book is available from the British Library.

Set in 10pt Times NR Monotype by Graphicraft Limited, Hong Kong

01   2009

Contents

List of Contributors

John Abraham
School of Social Sciences
University of Sussex
Brighton
Sussex, UK

Michael Barr
PEALS
University of Newcastle
Newcastle, UK

Sharon Boden
School of Criminology, Education,
Sociology and Social Work
Keele University
Keele
Staffordshire, UK

Laura M. Carpenter
Department of Sociology
Vanderbilt University
Nashville, USA

Monica Casper
Department of Sociology
Vanderbilt University
Nashville, USA

Fabian Cataldo
Department of Anthropology
Goldsmith's College
University of London
London, UK

Peter Conrad
Department of Sociology
Brandeis University
Massachusetts, USA

Peter Davis
Social Statistics Research Group
University of Auckland
Auckland, New Zealand

Catherine Duggan
Practice and Policy
School of Pharmacy
London, UK

Jonathan Gabe
Department of Health and
Social Care
Royal Holloway
University of London
Surrey, UK

Nick J. Fox
ScHARR
University of Sheffield
Sheffield, UK

Kathryn Jones
Department of Public Policy
De Montfort University
Leicester, UK

Valerie Leiter
Department of Sociology
Simmons College
Boston, Massachusetts, USA

Miranda Leontowitsch
Health and Social Care
St George's Medical School
London, UK

Pam Lowe
School of Languages and
Social Sciences
Aston University
Birmingham, UK

Mike Michael
Department of Sociology
Goldsmith's College
University of London
London, UK

Diana Rose
MHR Biomedical Research Centre
King's College London
London, UK

Clive Seale
Institute of Health Sciences
Queen Mary, University of London
London, UK

Deborah Lynn Steinberg
Department of Sociology
University of Warwick
Coventry, UK

Fiona A. Stevenson
Primary Care and Population
Sciences
University College London
London, UK

Steven P. Wainwright
Centre for Biomedicine and Society
King's College London
London, UK

Katie J. Ward
ScHARR
University of Sheffield
Sheffield, UK

Clare Williams
Centre for Biomedicine and Society
King's College London
London, UK

Simon J. Williams
Department of Sociology
University of Warwick
Coventry, UK

1

The sociology of pharmaceuticals: progress and prospects
Simon J. Williams, Jonathan Gabe and Peter Davis

Introduction

Recent years have witnessed an upsurge of interest in pharmaceuticals and society, a trend which in part reflects the growing power and influence of the pharmaceutical industry over all our lives, as patients, consumers and citizens. Medicine costs the National Health Service (NHS) in England alone over £7 billion every year, 80 per cent of which is spent on branded (patented) products, with the pharmaceutical industry the third most profitable activity in the UK economy after tourism and finance (House of Commons Health Committee 2005). These figures, in turn, are part and parcel of the bigger global picture of pharmaceuticals sales which are forecast to grow by five to six per cent between 2007 and 2008 to over US $735 billion a year – with North American sales alone constituting nearly half of this market, and North American and European pharmaceutical sales together constituting over three-quarters of global pharmaceutical sales (IMS MIDAS 2008 http:// www.imshealth.com). Scarcely a day goes by, moreover, without some story or other in the media about pharmaceutical products and practices. On the one hand, newspaper headlines boast new breakthrough 'wonder drugs'. On the other hand, stories of drug crises or controversies are regularly rehearsed in the media, thereby stirring fear and fascination in the public mind as to the power of pharmaceuticals and the industry that markets and manufactures them. Clearly pharmaceuticals have an important role to play in the alleviation of human suffering and the saving of lives. They are also, however, the source of much controversy, contestation and conflict, not simply in terms of their development, testing and marketing, but in terms of their very meaning and consumption.

This monograph is both a reflection of and response to this upsurge of interest in pharmaceuticals and society, casting further critical sociological light on these developments, discourses and debates. It is possible, in this respect, to point to a variety of themes and issues which taken together demonstrate both progress in sociological research on pharmaceuticals over the years and future prospects.

Medicalisation and pharmaceuticalisation; doctors, disorders and drugs

The first and perhaps most long-standing sociological theme has centred on the role of pharmaceuticals in the medicalisation of society. When Illich (1975), way back in the 1970s, talked of the iatrogenic effects of modern medicine and how the consumption of medical products helped sponsor a 'morbid society', a key target of his critique was our 'over-reliance' or 'dependence' on drugs as well as doctors. Others more fully or squarely located within medical sociology, particularly North American medical sociology, have also taken up these themes, albeit in a less radical or libertarian way than Illich. Specific emphasis has been placed by these authors on the expansion of medical jurisdiction and control over more and more areas of our lives, in the name of health and illness (Zola 1970, Freidson 1970, Conrad and Schneider 1980a,b). The role of the pharmaceutical industry within these processes, nonetheless, remained a somewhat muted or neglected theme in the medicalisation literature of the 1970s through to the 1990s, with sociological attention focusing on the power and influence of medicine in the social construction of disease and decisions about its treatment. More recent work, however, has begun to reappraise these processes in the light of current trends and developments regarding the medicalisation of society. Conrad (2005, 2007, Conrad and Leiter 2004), for example, in updating his previous work in this area (Conrad 1992, Conrad and Schneider 1980a,b), has pointed to what he terms the 'shifting engines' or 'drivers' of medicalisation over time – see also Clarke *et al.* (2003) for a somewhat different line or emphasis on transitions from medicalisation to so-called 'biomedicalisation'. Whilst the definitional centre of medicalisation remains with doctors, Conrad argues, the primary drivers of medicalisation now pertain to consumerism, managed care markets and developments in biotechnology, including the pharmaceutical industry.

Other more critical commentators (many of whom, significantly, are not sociologists), have taken these arguments one or more steps further, claiming that what may once have been regarded as medicalisation is now best seen as outright 'disease-mongering' in which the helping hand of the pharmaceutical industry looms large. Critics such as Moynihan (Moynihan 2002, Moynihan and Henry 2006, Moynihan *et al.* 2002) and Blech (2006), for example, through a series of case studies, have shown how pharmaceutical companies in collaboration or conjunction with doctors, pressure groups and the media, are no longer simply manufacturers of drugs but of diseases for these drugs to treat! – see also Law (2006) on 'Big Pharma'. A recent issue of the *Public Library of Science – Medicine*, for instance, devoted a whole section to essays on this very issue, including case studies of a range of diseases or disorders from ADHD (Phillips 2006) through erectile dysfunction (Lexchin 2006) and female sexual dysfunction (Tiefer 2006) to bipolar disorder (Healy 2006). These critiques, to be sure, are important. Not all forms of medicalisation, however, involve disease-mongering. Nor do all forms of medicalisation entail pharmaceuticals or processes of pharmaceuticalisation. Ideally, medicalisation should be considered as a value-neutral term that simply denotes the making or turning of something into a medical matter, the merits of which are open to empirical investigation depending on the case in question (Conrad 2007, 1992). Medicalisation, as such, may have positive and negative or light and dark faces, involving both gains and losses for the parties involved.

Whatever the merits of the case for outright disease mongering, one key vehicle for the expansion of pharmaceutical markets is of course direct-to-consumer advertising (DTCA): a development which to date is limited to countries such as the USA and New Zealand. On the one hand, this may be viewed as an entirely new development or departure. On the other hand, an instructive parallel and precursor may be found in the guise of patent medicine advertising in the past. Conrad and Leiter's chapter, for example, sheds valuable further light on these issues. Taking two advertising exemplars as its case studies – the late 19th century Lydia E. Pinkham's vegetable compounds for 'women's complaints' and contemporary Levitra for 'erectile dysfunction' (ED) – instructive parallels are drawn by these authors between the patent medicine era and the DTCA era. One of the great ironies of DTCA in this respect, Conrad and Leiter argue, is that it extends the relationship of drug companies, physicians and consumers in ways that rehearse or return us to a situation similar to Lydia Pinkham's day, when the drug manufacturers had a direct and independent relationship with consumers. Whilst the extravagant claims of Pinkham are now constrained by law, moreover, we must also contend with the fact that modern advertising has become far more subtle and sophisticated in its attempts to persuade or convince consumers that its products are the right ones in an increasingly competitive pharmaceutical marketplace. The pharmaceutical industry and consumers, Conrad and Leiter conclude, are increasingly important players in medicalisation, facilitated in part by the advent (or return to) DTCA.

Another key factor or player in these medicalising processes, of course, as Conrad and Leiter's chapter on DTCA clearly attests, are the media. Previous sociological studies, for example, have demonstrated both celebratory and critical media discourses on drugs, depending on the media, format and drug in question, the relative 'newness' of the drug to the market, and its 'newsworthiness'. For example, when benzodiazepine tranquillisers were first prescribed in the 1960s they generally received an enthusiastic welcome in the UK and US media and were proclaimed as heralding a new therapeutic era. As their popularity grew, however, their therapeutic value ceased to be newsworthy and a more critical coverage developed, drawing on the comments of a small but growing band of professional and lay critics. Initially, in the 1970s, this concern focused on claims about their overuse as a 'chemical crutch' for personal problems, before shifting in the 1980s and 1990s to claims about these drugs' 'addictive' potential, (Gabe and Bury 1996a, 1996b), with users portrayed in the local and national UK press as innocent victims, through no fault of their own, who then tried to withdraw and embark on a 'return journey' to normality (Gabe et al. 1991). Moreover, through these forms of mediation and marketing, drugs may come to take on personalities of their own, achieving some sort of quasi-mythic or celebrity status in the popular imagination, construed or constructed as the archetypal hero or villain (see for example Martin 2007, Nelkin 1995).

Some of these issues, for instance, are addressed in Williams and colleagues' chapter on newspaper coverage of the wakefulness-promoting drug Modafinil (brand name Provigil). Constructions of this drug in the print news media, these authors show, range from largely uncritical endorsement of its clinical applications as a 'breakthrough' or 'wonder drug' for a growing list of sleepiness-related conditions, to somewhat more cautious or critical coverage of its wider (potential) uptake as a lifestyle drug of choice, or in sport or military contexts. Again, we see here, in the guise of this wakefulness-promoting drug, the now familiar if not commonplace rehearsal of concern over the blurring or shifting boundaries between 'treatment' and 'enhancement', and the broader articulation of cultural anxieties about a move to a 24/7 society in which sleep becomes increasingly optional if not obsolete. A notable feature of the chapter, in this respect, is the authors' preference for the term 'pharmaceuticalisation' rather than medicalisation in order to capture these concerns in the press: concerns, that is to say, to do with the potentially widespread use and uptake of pharmaceuticals for diverse purposes which extend far beyond the realms of medicine or the strictly medical.

Another prime expression of the mediation of pharmaceuticals, of course, concerns the Internet or cyber-space/culture – see, for example, Miah and Rich (2008). This includes not simply access to information on pharmaceuticals via Internet searches, but the purchase of pharmaceuticals through online or e-pharmacies and the sharing of information and support through Internet chat rooms and online forums of various sorts (Fox et al. 2005a,b). In these and other ways, new opportunities for the mediation of pharmaceuticals are opening up in all our lives, for better or worse, routes that may very well bypass the traditional doctor-patient relationship altogether. Some of these issues, for example, are taken up in Fox and Ward's chapter on the pharmaceuticalisation of daily life – as with Williams et al.'s chapter, the preference for pharmaceuticalisation over medicalisation is once again notable. Taking as their problematic the new emphasis on lifestyle in the production, marketing and consumption of pharmceuticals and drawing on a diverse array of sources – including literature from social science, economics and health services research, together with their own research on pharmaceutical consumption – Fox and Ward identify two broad processes at work here. First, a domestication of pharmaceutical consumption, through computer mediated access and consumption within the home, particularly the bedroom and the kitchen. Second, the pharmaceuticalisation of everyday life, as pharmaceuticals come to be seen by consumers as 'magic bullets' for a range of everyday daily life problems. The domestication of pharmaceutical consumption and the pharmaceuticalisation of life, in this respect, become a complex mixture or heady brew of factors, including the biological effects of the drug on the body, the legitimacy of the problem or disorder in question, the willingness of consumers to adopt the technology as a 'solution' to a problem in their lives, and the corporate interests of the pharmaceutical industry. For these authors social relations surrounding contemporary pharmaceutical production and consumption 'link the world of business to the private world of citizens, forging new diseases and treatments from the very fabric of daily life'.

Regulation; science, politics and the pharmaceutical industry

If medicalisation and pharmaceuticalistion constitute one key strand of sociological research on pharmaceuticals and society over the years, then the science and politics of the pharmaceutical industry, including issues of development, testing and regulation, constitute another rich seam of work. Abraham (1993, 1995, 1997, 2002, 2007, Abraham and Davis 2005, Abraham and Lewis 2002, Abraham and Reed 2001, Abraham and Sheppard 1999), for example, has been at the forefront of this research over the past 15 to 20 years, documenting through detailed empirical case study work and comparative analysis elements of controversy and corporate 'bias' which, at one and the same time, demonstrate the inadequacies of existing regulatory practices and procedures, and the need for more rigorous and robust policy interventions at the institutional and legislative levels. These include the development of independent drugs testing by regulatory authorities, increased patient and public representation on regulatory committees and more frequent and thorough oversight of regulatory performance by the legislature – see also Busfield's (2007a) recent sociological analysis of scientific 'fact making' in the clinical trials of drugs and in post-approval drugs assessment, and the subsequent Abraham (2007)-Busfield (2007b) debate.

Many of these issues were explicitly taken up and addressed by the House of Commons Health Committee (2005) Report on *The Influence of the Pharmaceutical Industry*. Whilst rightly noting how pharmaceuticals may be a force for the good in contributing to the health of the nation, the report is nonetheless peppered with references to a 'failing' regulatory system, to 'lax oversight' and to practices on the part of the pharamaceutical industry which 'act against the public interest', given the power and influence of marketing forces. Recommendations cover several key areas, including the licensing process, with greater transparency and independent assessment of evidence, improved Medicine and Health Care Products Regulatory Agency (MHRA) mechanisms for restraints on medicines promotion, tougher restrictions and greater vigilance to guard against 'excessive' or 'inappropriate' prescribing, and a fundamental review of the MHRA itself.

In revisiting these issues, Abraham's chapter provides both a timely review of 20 years of sociological research on pharmaceutical development and regulation and a reassertion of the importance of a realist empirical research programme for the investigation of these issues, based on the notion of 'objective interests' – *i.e.* the objective interests of pharmaceutical companies in profit maximisation and the objective interests of patients/public health in the optimisation of the benefit-risk ratio of drugs. Drawing on international comparisons of drug regulation, Abraham shows how commercial interests have biased the science of drug testing and review away from patients and the public in favour of the industry: a process, he argues, which is best characterised as 'neo-liberal corporate bias'.

Far from being the 'inevitable by-product' of technoscientific progress in pharmaceuticals, moreover, these international comparisons are valuable in demonstrating considerable scope for improvement. Similarly, the lowering of technoscientific standards for drug safety across the EU, US and Japan is not, Abraham argues, an inevitable price to be paid for faster development of therapeutically valuable medicines, but more plausibly a consequence of the international spread of neo-liberal corporate bias in pharmaceutical regulation.

The gender and sexual politics of pharmaceutical development, testing, and regulation adds another important dimension to the picture here. We see this very clearly, for example, in Casper and Carpenter's chapter on the politics and controversy surrounding initiatives to introduce the human papilloma virus (HPV) vaccine for cervical cancer in the United States of America. These initiatives have, in the words of the authors, 'animated longstanding concerns about vaccination . . . and young women's bodies and behavior'. The HPV vaccine, in this respect, raises the spectre of both past controversies about vaccination and current political concerns in the area of sexual morality. Vaccines, the authors argue, are a distinctive kind of pharmaceutical invoking notions of 'contagion' and 'containment'. Pharmaceuticals, moreover, develop lives or biographies of their own; trajectories shaped at every stage or phase by politics. Viewed in this light then, it is not so much the public debates about vaccination as such that are the most important dimensions to the story here, but that its target is a sexually-transmitted disease, which thereby draws into the debate issues of sex, gender and women's bodies that are far more charged. The launch of the HPV vaccine in short, these authors argue, appears to have 'inflamed' US health care politics which in turn has affected plans for marketing the drug. This in turn underlines both the struggles provoked by this new gendered technology and the ever emerging and evolving 'biographies' of pharmaceuticals themselves, which to repeat, are deeply political.

Broader questions also arise at this point about the global nature and dynamics of the pharmaceutical industry. These include debates on the 'globalisation' of medicines control (Abraham and Reed 2003), whether or not the pharmaceutical industry is in fact truly 'globalised' in the first place – multinationalisation, or Westernisation, Busfield (2003) argues, are more accurate terms of reference – and the growing practice of out-sourcing or 'pharming' out clinical trials to the developing world where regulatory standards are lower or looser and bodies are in cheap supply (Shah 2007). Important questions need to be asked here, for example, about who gets what, when, and where - *i.e.* the global inequalities and injustices spawned through the current system of drugs development and distribution. Of particular significance here is the prioritisation of drugs for affluent societies where chronic conditions prevail and lucrative markets beckon over other basic life-saving drugs for those in poorer parts of the world, many of whom exist on less than a dollar a day (Busfield 2007a, Petryna *et al.* 2006, Shah 2007).

One seeming success story on this count, at face value at least, concerns the state-sponsored national provision of Antiretroviral Therapy (ART) for people with HIV in Brazil. Yet, as Cataldo's chapter suggests, based on his detailed ethnographic research in a *favela* (shanty town) in Brazil, the universal character of this public health programme is challenged or problematised in a number of ways through local definitions of illness, problems of adherence to treatment, structural violence, political alienation and the lack of perspectives about the future. These developments, moreover, echoing other writers (Petryna 2002, Petryna *et al.* 2006, Biehl 2004, Rose 2007), point to new or novel forms of socio-political identification and participation focused on the notion of 'therapeutic' or 'biological citizenship'. In particular, they raise concerns about free access to treatment, the right to health care, and the viability and sustainability of public health policies in a 'developing' or 'middle income' country.

Consumption and consumerism; medicines in the marketplace

A third long-standing strand of sociological research on pharmaceuticals concerns what may loosely be termed consumption and consumerism. Initial work in this area focused on providing a 'social audit' of the use of prescribed medicines in the community (*e.g.* Dunnell and Cartwright 1972). In the 1980s and 1990s the focus shifted to exploring the social meaning of medications ranging from anti-hypertensives (Morgan 1996) to benzodi-azepine tranquillisers (Helman 1981, Gabe and Lipshitz-Phillips 1982, 1984, Gabe and Thorogood 1986) and how such meanings were shaped by users' ethnicity and gender (Cooperstock and Lennard 1979, Gabe and Thorogood 1986, Ettorre and Riska 1995).

More recently, with the growing sociological interest in consumption and consumerism (Rief 2008), attention has increasingly focused on users of pharmaceuticals as knowledge-able and reflexive actors, assessing the risks and benefits and making informed choices in consultation with professionals (Fox *et al.* 2007, Fox *et al.* 2005a). Such consumerism, in turn, is reinforced by UK government policy which constructs patients as experts and exhorts professionals to develop a 'partnership' with their patients (Taylor and Bury 2007). These developments are explored in the chapter by Stevenson, Leontowitsch and Duggan, who consider how consumers of over-the-counter medicines engage with pharmacists, and how pharmacists seek to maintain their professional expertise in the face of health-care consumerism. Based on interviews with customers and pharmacists, group discussions with pharmacists and tape-recorded consultations and observations in two pharmacies, they show how pharmacists' attempts to engage customers in discussions about their treatment did not result in a reduction in the importance of pharmaceutical expertise. Instead, both pharmacists and customers acknowledged the importance of the asymmetry of knowledge between them. Nonetheless, customers did not always see pharmaceutical expertise to be necessary and at times talked about over-the-counter medicines as a commodity, and treated transactions in pharmacies as no different from those in other retail outlets. And pharmacists were aware that they were running a business and that they needed to be sensitive to the danger of losing trade if they resisted selling a product that a customer had requested.

Sociological work on consumerism is not just focused on individual users of health care as knowledgeable and reflexive actors. Attention has also been paid to the way in which users act collectively to represent their interests as members of self-help groups, patient-advocacy groups and health social movements in the public sphere (Kelleher 2004, Brown *et al.* 2004). In the case of pharmaceuticals this has involved focusing on how health consumer groups – voluntary sector organisations that represent the interests of patients – engage with the pharmaceutical industry around issues such as the availability of and access to medicines. This provides the focus for the chapter by Jones. She explores how health consumer groups in the UK disclose and manage links with pharmaceutical companies in the context of their increasing involvement in the policy process. She focuses on claims that companies engage with groups in order to try and 'capture' their policy agenda. Drawing on evidence from group and industry websites and interviews with representatives of consumer groups, industry and other health-care stakeholders she reveals that only around a quarter of groups known to receive financial or in-kind support openly admit to this. Even so, Jones rejects the view that this lack of transparency demonstrates that these groups' policy agenda has been 'captured'. Rather, she points to a coincidence of aims (both sides have an interest in medicines being available), the existence of tacit support for guidelines to manage conflicts and the fact that funding from industry generally represents only a small proportion of these groups' income. Nonetheless she acknowledges that the lack of transparency with regard to disclosing funding strengthens critiques of undue influence and may well reduce policy makers' willingness to treat consumer groups as the legitimate voice of patients in the policy process.

Expectations and innovation; pharmacogenomics, regenerative medicine and beyond ...

A fourth and final strand of sociological research has been very much taken up with innovative new developments in bioscience, biomedicine and biotechnology, including pharmaceuticals, which, taken together, point to or promise reconfigured futures. Rose (2007), for example, in his broad survey of this newly emerging field, highlights what he takes to be the growing 'politicisation' of all life forms, given the rapid pace of developments in bioscience, biotechnology and biomedicine at the dawn of the 21st century. This politicisation covers the morphing or mutating of biomedicine through molecularisation, debates around the very nature and status of what it is to be 'human', the formation of new biosocial identities, communities and forms of citizenship, and the reconfiguration of the boundaries between normality and abnormality, health and illness, treatment and enhancement. Developments in neuroscience, for example, including novel forms of psychopharmacological intervention or enhancement, raise a host of social, legal, ethical, political and economic issues which necessitate informed dialogue and debate across disciplinary boundaries and wider public and policy-making arenas – see, for example, the recent flurry of reports on cognitive enhancement agents by the Academy of Medical Sciences (2008), British Medical Association (2007), Department of Trade and Industry (2005). Psychopharmaceuticals, in this respect, are becoming central to the way in which conduct is governed, obliging individuals to engage in 'constant risk management, to monitor and evaluate mood, emotion, cognition, according to finer and more continuous processes of self-scrutiny' (Rose 2007: 223).

These developments in turn encourage us to ask pertinent sociological questions about the biopolitics of the future, including sociology's own role in the co-construction or co-production of various utopian and dystopian biofutures. Recent research on the sociology of *expectations*, for example, has drawn attention to: (i) the dynamic role which expectations play in defining roles, attracting investors and building mutually binding obligations; (ii) how expectations differ between various social groups (*e.g.* scientists, policy communities, industry, consumers, public); and (iii) how the futures they envisage are 'contingent', 'contested', 'embraced', 'imagined', including both the 'retrospecting of prospects' and the 'prospecting of retrospects' (Brown and Michael 2003) – see also Novas (2001) on the political economy of hope.

The development of new vaccines, for example, is an obvious case in point, generating hopes, fears, and a variety of other moral and political agendas which both hark back to the past and project into the future – see, for example, Casper and Carpenter's chapter discussed above. Another key area where these issues are very clearly evident is in relation to recent developments in pharmacogenetics and pharmacogenomics (*i.e.* the splicing or hybridisation of pharmacological and genetic/genomic knowledge in order to predict drug reactions). This is a field of considerable hyperbole and hope regarding a new era of so-called 'personalised', 'bespoke' or 'tailor-made' medicines, construed as the perfect antidote to the 'one-size-fits-all' remedies currently on the market, where side-effects or adverse drug reactions (ADRs) are commonplace. Whilst major pharmaceutical industry interest and investment in this area is relatively recent (little more than 10 years old in fact), pharmacogenetics as a term of reference or organising principle has been around much longer, dating back to the late 1950s. These developments, moreover, generate a number of concerns from a diverse range of constituencies, including potential problems of 'over-segmented' (read 'unprofitable') markets, the proliferation of genetic testing, and the 'racial politics' of personalised medicine – see Brown and Webster (2004), and Sneddon (2000) for useful discussions of some of these issues and Hedgecoe (2004) for an illuminating study of the politics of pharmcogenetics in relation to Alzheimer's and breast cancer. Questions also arise as to just how personalised these developments can ever be. To the extent indeed that 'personalised' medicine is ever truly possible, then as Hedgecoe (2004: 5) wryly remarks, this is best seen as the equivalent of purchasing a small, medium or large T-shirt from GAP than of being fitted for a smart tailor-made Savile Row suit!

Barr and Rose's chapter sheds further comparative light on some of these issues in relation to anti-depressant drugs. Drawing on their empirical study of the views of patients with depression regarding genome-based therapies for their condition (GENDEP) in eight European countries – England, Poland, Slovenia, Italy, Belgium Denmark, Germany and Croatia – these authors show how discussions of the clinical acceptability of genome-based therapies for depression cannot be divorced from some of the wider issues regarding depression and anti-depressants. This includes a commonplace tendency to conflate notions of a pharmacogenomic test for antidepressants with a genetic test for depression, doubts about the medical model of depression, and a 'deep ambivalence' regarding the use of anti-depressant medication. On the one hand, strong hope is expressed about new drugs to treat depression. On the other hand, concerns remain over the need to take such drugs either now or in the future to manage or modify moods. These views in turn are tied up with a belief that psychiatric illness is somehow 'different' from physical illness and that depression carries with it a certain cultural value, including positive links to creativity, selfhood and identity. There is then, in short, as these authors clearly demonstrate, a great 'ambivalence' regarding the personal and cultural significance accorded to depression and anti-depressant medications which genetic testing is likely to exacerbate rather than alleviate.

Another key area of hyperbole and hope concerns current research into stem cells: developments which hold out the promise or prospects of new treatments for conditions such as Alzheimer's disease, Parkinson's disease and motor neurone disease, through the cultivation of replacement neurons. At first glance this may have seemingly little to do with pharmaceutical investments, signifying in fact a direct threat or challenge to prevailing drug-based forms of treatment in the present or future, personalised or otherwise. Yet, as Wainwright and colleagues' chapter in this monograph suggests, a new paradigm of stem cells research is emerging, the 'disease in a dish' approach, whereby human embryonic stem cells (hESC) will be used as 'tools' to unravel the mechanisms of disease and enable the development of new drugs. It is here, at this nexus of regenerative medicine, hESC and pharmaceuticals, that a new set of problems and expectations is being forged; developments which Wainwright and colleagues argue can profitably be understood in terms of Bourdieu's theoretical concepts of capital, habitus and field, particularly 'expectational capital' which is derived from this set of ideas. Experts' persuasion practices and strategies, from this perspective, advance their interests in this uncertain field; a performative strategy which helps stabilise this emerging 'disease in a dish' model of translational research and new pharmaceutical drug development.

Taken together then, a variety of sociological agendas, both old and new, coalesce around pharmaceuticals and society, as this introduction clearly attests; issues, to repeat, which touch all our lives as patients, consumers and citizens. At a time of reinvigorated debate about the political and public faces of sociology (Burawoy 2005, Turner 2004), and the biopolitics of life itself (Rose 2007), sociological research on pharmaceuticals holds out the potential, promise or prospect of analyses which combine an appreciation of what

Wright Mills (1959), in the *Sociological Imagination*, classically described as personal troubles and broader public issues of social structure. In potentially holding those in positions of power to account, moreover, and in engaging in informed dialogue and debate with its publics, sociological research on pharmaceuticals admirably demonstrates the continuing importance of the discipline to these developments, discourses and debates. The contributions gathered together in this monograph, we believe, exemplify this promise and potential in an era where the power and force of pharmaceuticals to treat or enhance us, and the interests shaping their development and distribution, manufacture and marketing, look set to grow well into the 21st century.

References

Abraham, J. (1993) Scientific standards and institutional interests: carcinogenic risk assessment for Benoxaprofen in the UK and the US, *Social Studies of Science*, 23, 387–444.

Abraham, J. (1995) *Science, Politics and the Pharmaceutical Industry: Controversy and Bias in Drug Regulation*. London: UCL Press.

Abraham, J. (1997) The science and politics of medicines regulation. In Elston, M.A. (ed.) *Sociology of Health and Illness Special Monograph Issue on the Sociology of Medical Science and Technology*. Oxford: Blackwell.

Abraham, J. (2002) The pharmaceutical industry as a political player, *Lancet*, 360, 1498–502.

Abraham, J. (2007) Building on sociological understandings of the pharmaceutical industry or reinventing the wheel? Responses to Joan Busfield's 'Pills, power and people', *Sociology*, 41, 727–36.

Abraham, J. and Davis, C. (2005) A comparative analysis of drug safety withdrawals in the UK and the US (1971–1992): implications for current regulatory thinking and policy, *Social Science and Medicine*, 61, 881–92.

Abraham, J. and Lewis, G. (2002) Citizenship, medical expertise and the regulatory state in Europe, *Sociology*, 36, 1, 67–88.

Abraham, J. and Reed, T. (2001) Trading risks for markets: the international harmonisation of pharmaceuticals regulation, *Health, Risk and Society: Special issue on Globalisation*, 3, 113–28.

Abraham, J. and Reed, T. (2003) Globalization of medicines control. In Abraham, J. and Lawton Smith, H. (eds) *Regulation of the Pharmaceutical Industry*. Basingstoke: Palgrave.

Abraham, J. and Sheppard, J. (1999) *Therapeutic Nightmare: The Battle of the World's most Controversial Sleeping Pill*. London: Earth Scan.

Academy of Medical Sciences (2008) *Brain Science, Addictions and Drugs*. London: AMS.

Biehl, J. (2004) The activist state: global pharmaceuticals, AIDS and citizenship in Brazil, *Social Texts*, 22, 3, 105–32.

Blech, J. (2006) *Inventing Diseases and Pushing Pills: Pharmaceutical Companies and the Medicalisation of Normal Life*. London: Routledge.

British Medical Association (2007) *Boosting Your Brain Power: Ethical Aspects of Cognitive Enhancements*. London: BMA.

Brown, N. and Michael, M. (2003) A sociology of expectations: retrospecting prospects and prospecting retrospects, *Technology Assessment and Strategic Management*, 15, 1, 3–18.

Brown, N. and Webster, A. (2004) *New Medical Technologies and Society*. Cambridge: Polity Press.

Brown, P., Zavestoski, S., McCormick, S., Mayer, B., Morello-Frosch, R. and Altman, R. (2004) Embodied health movements: new approaches to social movements in health, *Sociology of Health and Illness*, 26, 50–80.

Buroway, M. (2005) American presidential address: for public sociology, *British Journal of Sociology*, 56, 2, 259–94.

Busfield, J. (2003) Globalization and the pharmaceutical industry revisited, *International Journal of Health Services*, 33, 3, 581–603.

Busfield, J. (2007a) Pills, power and people: sociological understandings of the pharmaceutical industry, *Sociology*, 40, 297–314.

Busfield, J. (2007b) Sociological understandings of the pharmaceutical industry: a response to John Abraham, *Sociology*, 41, 737–39.

Clarke, A., Fishman, J., Fosket, J.R., Mamo, L. and Shim, J. (2003) Biomedicalization: Technoscientific transformations of health, illness, and US biomedicine, *American Sociological Review*, 68, 161–94.

Conrad, P. (1992) Medicalisation and social control, *Annual Review of Sociology*, 18, 209–32.

Conrad, P. (2005) The shifting engines of medicalization, *Journal of Health and Social Behavior*, 46, 3–14.

Conrad, P. (2007) *The Medicalisation of Society*. Baltimore: Johns Hopkins University Press.

Conrad, P. and Leiter, V. (2004) Medicalization, markets and consumers, *Journal of Health and Social Behavior*, 45, 158–76.

Conrad, P. and Schneider, J. (1980a) *Deviance and Medicalization: from Badness to Sickness*. St Louis: Mosby.

Conrad, P. and Schneider, J. (1980b) Looking at levels of medicalisation: a comment on Strong's critique of the thesis of medical imperialism, *Social Science and Medicine*, 14, 75–9.

Cooperstock, R. and Lennard, H. (1979) Some social meanings of tranquilliser use, *Sociology of Health and Illness*, 1, 2, 238–44.

Department of Trade and Industry (Office of Science and Technology) (2005) *Drugs Futures 2025*. London: DTI.

Dunnell, K. and Cartwright, A. (1972) *Medicine-takers, Prescribers and Hoarders*. London: Routledge and Kegan Paul.

Ettorre, E. and Riska, E. (1995) *Gendered Moods. Psychotropics and Society*. London: Routledge.

Fox, N.J., Ward, K.J. and O'Rourke, A.J. (2005a) The 'expert pateint': empowerment or medical dominance? The case of weight loss, phamaceutical drugs and the Internet, *Social Science and Medicine*, 60, 1299–309.

Fox, N.J., Ward, K.J. and O'Rourke, A.J. (2005b) Pro-Anorexia, weight-loss drugs and the Internet: an 'anti-recovery' explanatory model of anorexia, *Sociology of Health and Illness*, 27, 2, 944–71.

Fox, N.J., Ward, K.J. and O'Rourke, A.J. (2007) A sociology of technology governance for the information age: the case of pharmaceuticals, consumer advertising and the Internet, *Sociology*, 40, 315–34.

Freidson, E. (1970) *Professional Dominance*. New York: Dodds Mead.

Gabe, J. and Lipshitz-Phillips, S. (1982) Evil necessity? The meaning of benzodiazepine use for women patients from one general practice, *Sociology of Health and Illness*, 4, 201–9.

Gabe, J. and Lipshitz-Phillips, S. (1984) Tranquillisers as social control? *Sociological Review*, 32, 524–46.

Gabe, J. and Thorogood, N. (1986) Prescribed drug use and the management of everyday life: the experiences of black and white working class women, *Sociological Review*, 34, 737–72.

Gabe, J. and Bury, M. (1996a) Halcion nights: a sociological account of a medical controversy, *Sociology*, 30, 447–69.

Gabe, J. and Bury, M. (1996b) Risking tranquilliser use: cultural and lay dimensions. In Williams, S. and Calnan, M. (eds) *Modern Medicine. Lay Perspectives and Experiences*. London: UCL Press.

Gabe, J., Gustafsson, U. and Bury, M. (1991) Mediating illness: newspaper coverage of tranquilliser dependence, *Sociology of Health and Illness*, 13, 4, 332–53.

Harding, G. and Taylor, K. (1997) Responding to change: the case of community pharmacy in Britain, *Sociology of Health and Illness*, 19, 5, 547–60.

Healy, D. (2006) The latest mania: selling biopolar disorder, *Public Library of Science – Medicine*, 3, 4, e. 185.

Hedgecoe, A. (2004) *The Politcs of Personalised Medicine*. Cambridge: Cambridge University Press.

Helman, C. (1981) 'Tonic', 'fuel' and 'food': social and symbolic aspects of the long term use of psychotropic drugs, *Social Science and Medicine*, 15B, 521–33.

Hibbert, D., Bissell, P. and Ward, P. (2002) Consumerism and professional work in the community pharmacy, *Sociology of Health and Illness*, 24, 1, 46–65.

House of Commons Health Committee (2005) *The Influence of the Pharmaceutical Industry* (Fourth Report for Session 2004–5). London: The Stationary Office Ltd.

Illich, I. (1975) *Medical Nemesis*. London: Marion Boyars.

Kelleher, D. (2004) Self help groups and their relationship to medicine. In Kelleher, D., Gabe, J. and Williams, G. (eds) (2004) *Challenging Medicine*, 2nd Edition. London: Routledge.

Law, J. (2006) *The Big Pharma*. London: Constable and Robinson.

Lexchin, J. (2006) Bigger and better: how Pfizer redefined erectile dysfunction, *Public Library of Science – Medicine*, 3, 4, e. 132.

Martin, E. (2007) *Bipolar*. Princeton: Princeton University Press.

Miah, A. and Rich, E. (2008) *The Medicalization of Cyberspace*. London: Routledge.

Mills, C.W. (1959) *The Sociological Imagination*. Oxford: Oxford University Press.

Morgan, M. (1996) Perceptions and use of anti-hypertensive drugs among cultural groups. In Williams, S. and Calnan, M. (eds) *Modern Medicine. Lay Perspectives and Experiences*. London: UCL Press.

Moynihan, R. (2002) Disease-mongering: how doctors, drug companies, and insurers are making you feel sick. *British Medical Journal*, 324, 923.

Moynihan, R. and Henry, D. (2006) The fight against disease mongering: generating knowledge for action, *Public Library of Science – Medicine*, 3, 4, e. 191.

Moynihan, R., Health, I. and Henry, D. (2002) Selling sickness: the pharmaceutical industry and disease mongering, *British Medical Journal*, 324, 886–91.

Nelkin, D. (1995) *Selling Science: how the Press Covers Science and Technology*. New York: W.H. Freeman.

Novas, C. (2001) The political economy of hope: patients' organisations, science and biovalue, *Bio-Societies*, 1, 3, 289–305.

Petryna, A. (2002) *Life Exposed: Biological Citizens after Chernobyl*. Princeton: Princeton University Press.

Petryna, A., Lakoff, A. and Kleinman, A. (eds) (2006) *Global Pharmaceuticals: Ethics, Markets, Practices*. Durham and London; Duke University Press.

Phillips, C.B. (2006) Medicine goes to school: teachers as sickness brokers for ADHD, *Public Library of Science – Medicine*, 3, 4, e. 182.

Rief, S. (2008) Outline of a critical sociology of consumption: beyond moralism and celebration, *Sociology Compass*, 2, 1–17.

Rose, N. (2007) *The Politics of Life Itself*. Princeton: Princeton University Press.

Shah, S. (2007) *Body Hunters: Testing New Drugs on the World's Poorest Patients*. London/New York: The New Press.

Sneddon, R. (2000) The challenge of pharmacogenetics and pharmacogenomics, *New Genetics and Society*, 19, 145–64.

Taylor, D. and Bury, M. (2007) Chronic illness, expert patients and care transition, *Sociology of Health and Illness*, 29, 1, 27–45.

Tiefer, L. (2006) Female sexual dysfunction: a case study of disease mongering and activist resistance, *Public Library of Science – Medicine*, 3, 4, e. 178.

Turner, B.S. (2004) *The New Medical Sociology*. London/NY: W.W. Norton and Co.

Zola, I.K. (1972) Medicine as an institution of social control, *Sociological Review*, 20, 487–503.

2

From Lydia Pinkham to Queen Levitra: direct-to-consumer advertising and medicalisation
Peter Conrad and Valerie Leiter

Introduction

The medicalisation of life problems has been occurring for well over a century (Conrad and Schneider 1992, Shorter 1992, Wertz and Wertz 1989) and may have increased in the past 30 years (Conrad 2005, 2007). Medicalisation occurs when previously non-medical problems are defined and treated as medical problems, usually in terms of illnesses or disorders, or when a medical intervention is used to treat the problem. In a recent article we argued that the push towards medicalisation comes more from the creation of medical markets than from professionals' desire to expand their jurisdiction (Conrad and Leiter 2004). Conrad (2005) has recently suggested that the shifting engines of medicalisation include biotechnology, managed care, and consumers.

In this chapter we examine one strand of medicalisation over the last century and a half: the role of direct-to-consumer advertising (DTCA) in the medicalisation of life problems. To do this we compare patent medicine advertising with contemporary DTCA, highlighting the role of federal regulation of pharmaceuticals and advertising as a constraint on medicalisation during the 20th century. We rely primarily upon secondary data sources plus some primary Congressional documents on DTCA in our analyses. This historical comparison allows us to analyse current DTCA practices not as a new development, but as hearkening back to the patent medicine era, and to analyse the role that the medical profession played in creating and maintaining constraints on the advertisement of pharmaceuticals. Lydia E. Pinkham's Vegetable Compound was an exemplar of advertising in its time, and erectile dysfunction drugs, including Levitra, are exemplars of the contemporary DTCA era. History is often a great relativiser. By contrasting drugs that were promoted 130 years apart we seek to reflect more clearly on the potentials and pitfalls of DTCA in the 21st century.

Patent medicines in the 19th century

It is important to recall the context of medicine in the 19th century. For example, in the US medicine was not a particularly prestigious profession, with often poorly trained practitioners and extremely limited medical knowledge. When the American Medical Association (AMA) was organised in 1847, among its goals were the improvement of the image of medicine and gaining control over the licensing of physicians (Freidson 1970). The public was ambivalent about the invasive and heroic medicine that most physicians offered, and hospitals were seen as places to go to die. In many communities in America there were no trained physicians, so self-help was an important alternative to medical care. One sector of medical care was so-called 'patent medicines'.

Medicines could be divided between 'ethical' drugs of known composition and patent drugs of undeclared composition. After the Civil War, there was a growing division between ethical drug firms and patent medicine firms (Spillane 2004). The ethical drug firms attempted to distance themselves from patent medicine firms and to align themselves with the fledgling medical profession by adopting the AMA code of not advertising directly to the public (Starr 1982). 'Indeed, the ethical firms took great pains to publicise the fact that they did not make direct advertising appeals to the general public, but confined their sales pitches to persuading doctors and druggists of the superiority and reliability of their brands' (Spillane 2004: 2).

Patent medicines in the US originated in Britain and were imported until entrepreneurs discovered the potential domestic market (Young 1961). They were not actually patented but were proprietary drugs with secret or unlisted formulations, with a copyrighted trademark. Patent medicines were advertised directly to the public, encouraging consumers to medicalise everyday symptoms, such as being tired or nervous, through self-diagnosis and self-medication. By the 1850s 'the medicine taking habit was instilled by large usage in the American people. People wanted to take something and many doctors prescribed to demand' (Young 1961: 158). Patent medicines were advertised widely in Britain as well. For example, Thomas Holloway, a patent medicine merchant and later philanthropist, in 1880 spent 50,000 pounds, a great sum at the time, on advertising nostrums that made him wealthy but were later deemed to have little medicinal value (Harrison-Barbet 1994).

There were no limits on what manufacturers or sellers could claim; it was caveat emptor for consumers. At first, cure-alls of the snake oil variety were promoted but manufacturers soon discovered that marketing drugs for specific ailments was more profitable (Applegate 1998). Most of these nostrums were promoted with wildly excessive claims as cures for cancer or arthritis, remedies for baldness or small busts, or restorers of manhood. Almost any possible problem could yield to patent medicine cures.

Advertising for patent medicines went directly from the manufacturer to the consumer. The invention of cheap pulp paper for newsprint helped create an important route for patent medicine advertising. Nostrum advertising accounted for nearly one-third of profits in the newspaper business. 'In 1847, 2000 newspapers ran 11 million medicine ads' (Anderson 2000: 38). By the 1870s, a quarter of all advertising was for proprietary drugs. Dr. James C. Ayer pioneered saturation advertising for his best-selling Cherry Pectoral, by running ads in every newspaper in the US (Anderson 2000: 41).

Ads often emphasised symptoms most people experienced (*e.g.* fatigue, pains, indigestion, sleeplessness, headaches), contributing to a cultural medicalisation of life problems. These drug companies borrowed from the rising prestige of medicine while at the same time distancing themselves from doctors, advertising their treatments as cheaper, safer, less brutal and quicker. Nostrum advertisers 'recognised that nearly every man (sic) is vulnerable to the power of suggestion and sought to make him sick so they could make him well'. (Young 1961: 184). As one analyst suggests, 'Medicine manufacturers didn't collect orders and then fill them, as was the practice with other goods. Rather, they created a steady supply of the product, and then generated the demand' (Anderson 2000: 11). By the early 20th century Americans shelled out $75 million a year, which translates into $1.6 billion in current buying power for patent medicines (Crossen 2004: B1). Patent medicines were at their zenith at the turn of the century, with over 28,000 nostrums, few as successful or well known as Lydia E. Pinkham's Vegetable Compound (Young 1961).

Lydia E. Pinkham's Vegetable Compound
After the financial 'panic' of 1873, the 54-year-old Lydia Pinkham, an abolitionist and school teacher, saw a business opportunity. She added ingredients to a herbal formula that her husband had received as part of a settlement for a debt and made it into a proprietary medicine, which she brewed and bottled in her cellar in Lynn, Massachusetts. Two years later, upon the advice of her son, she began marketing her product as Lydia E. Pinkham's

Vegetable Compound for 'women's weaknesses,' including menstrual cramps. Lydia's motto was 'Only a woman understands women's ills' (Pinkus: 2002). The compound had a pungent odour and a sharp aftertaste, and is thought to have contained black cohosh (roots and stems of a perennial herb), fenugreek seed, and at least 18 per cent alcohol (as a preservative, because Pinkham was a temperance supporter).

Pinkham was a pioneer in DTCA. After placing an elaborate first page newspaper ad in the *Boston Herald* in 1876, sales of the product rose significantly, and Pinkham became convinced of the value of advertising. In 1879, her son suggested that she place a likeness of herself on the label, replete with her grandmotherly features. Sales of her product increased dramatically and her picture became one of the most well known female images in print at the time (Simmons 2002). She encouraged women to write to her in confidence for counsel, and answered their letters, a service which continued even after her death in 1883. These letters offered sterling testimonials of the product's efficacy.

Over the years, more maladies were added to the advertisements. For example, an 1887 ad in the *New York Times* proclaimed:

> LYDIA E. PINKHAM'S VEGETABLE COMPOUND Offers the SUREST REMEDY for the PAINFUL ILLS AND DISORDERS SUFFERED BY WOMEN EVERYWHERE. It relieves pain, promotes regular and healthy reoccurrence of periods and is a great help to young girls and women past maturity. It strengthens the back and the pelvic organs, bringing relief and comfort to tired women who stand all day in home, shop and factory.
>
> Leucorrhea, Inflammation, Ulceration and Displacements of the Uterus have been cured by it, as women everywhere gratefully testify. Regular physicians often prescribe it. Sold by all Druggists $1.00 (cited in Applegate 1998: 80).

Lydia Pinkham's advertising to consumers was innovative and ubiquitous. Her Vegetable Compound was everywhere; her face was on labels, in newspaper ads, on fences in rural America, on trading cards, and in drug store displays. Very few nostrums had such wide recognition. In 1912 sales exceeded $1 million. In 1914, in response to federal regulation, the company changed the formula to remove the alcohol so it would not be taxed as an alcoholic beverage and modified its claims about effectiveness (Applegate 1998). After 1925 or so, sales of the product declined. The patent medicine companies' DTCA had been wildly successful for some companies but, increasingly, it was opposed by the medical profession and other articulate critics.

Campaigns against patent medicines and DTCA

In Paul Starr's (1982: 128) words, 'The nostrum makers were the nemesis of physicians'. They competed with physicians for medical business, offered supposedly safer but unproven 'cures', and undercut the authority of medicine. Patent medicines, with secret formulas and advertising to the public, posed a threat to physicians' still fledgling professional aspirations. Both patent medicines and physicians grew in popularity and use in the late 19th century. In fact, despite the competition, physicians also used patent medicines in their practices; by one count, in 1874 one per cent of physicians used patient medicines, increasing to over 20 per cent by 1902 (Starr 1982: 130). By another count, 90 per cent of doctors were prescribing proprietary medicines (Young 1961: 160).

The medical profession's concern about patent medicines manifested itself in a variety of campaigns against the industry. In 1900 the AMA started a campaign 'to make the "legitimate proprietary drugs" respond to the ethics of medicine', which included disclosing formulas and not advertising directly to the public (Starr 1982: 129). The AMA announced it would stop taking patent medicine advertisements around this time, then relaxed their standards for revenues' sake. As Young notes, 'In 1905, JAMA did not have as many bad ads as many medical journals, but that is only faint praise' (1961: 207). Medical journals and newspapers continued to rely on patent medicine advertising as a major source of revenue.

In 1906, the AMA set standards for both advertising and prescribing medications with the publication of *New and Nonofficial Remedies* (Starr 1982: 131). Drugs were not accepted if their manufacturers made false advertising claims, refused to disclose their drugs' composition, advertised directly to the public, or whose 'label, package or circular listed the diseases for which the drug was used' (Starr 1982: 132). Ethical drug companies had a 'gentleman's agreement' with physicians, under which physicians would legitimise the drugs with the 'ethical' label and the drug companies would acknowledge physicians' authority to diagnose illness and determine treatments. This agreement did not guarantee that drugs were safe, as ethical drugs might contain poisons such as arsenic. Rather, the term 'ethical' meant that the drug companies would be honest about the contents of their wares, would not knowingly make fraudulent claims about their efficacy, and would not bypass physicians' authority. The line was drawn. Companies could advertise to physicians only or they could not advertise to physicians at all. Despite losing revenues, newspapers began to cut back on DTCA for drugs that the AMA listed as fraudulent.

Muck-raking journalists were also on the case of exposing useless potions that were sold in the name of health. In 1903 the *Ladies Home Journal* published an exposé on the dangers of patent medicines. Samuel Hopkins Adams' in-depth investigative series, 'The Great American Fraud', published in *Colliers Weekly* in 1905, really made the public case against patent medicines. The articles named specific names and identified specific false promises and deceptions made in patent medicine advertising. The writers and editors of these magazines advocated for federal regulation on the promotion and sale of patent medicines (Applegate 1998).

Some states had already considered regulating patent medicines, but they were 'easily outmatched by the well funded lobby of the Proprietary Association of America' (Crossen 2004). The AMA distributed 150,000 copies of these articles from 1905 to 1910 (Starr 1982: 130). Adams' investigation, along with Upton Sinclair's *The Jungle*, a muckraking exposé of the meat packing industry, the AMA's campaign against nostrum marketing, and scientist and crusader Harvey W. Wiley's work with Congress, finally resulted in the Pure Food and Drug Act of 1906, the first federal legislation to control drugs and medications.

Federal regulation and drug advertising

The Act put constraints on advertising and marketing, stating that manufacturers had to print accurate ingredients on the label, they could not make false or exaggerated claims on the label, and that drugs had to meet certain standards of purity. As one indicator of the Act's impact, the 1897 Sears Roebuck catalogue had 17 out of 770 pages dedicated to the 'Drug Department'; the 1908 catalogue had fewer than two pages of 1200 on drugs (Isreal 1968 cited in Pinkus 2002). The federal law was amended in 1912 to include claims of effectiveness and in 1920 to cover newspaper advertising (Starr 1982: 132). By 1915, Lydia

E. Pinkham's Vegetable Compound had to cease advertising specifically for women's disorders and instead made the innocuous claim, 'Recommended as a Vegetable Tonic in conditions for which the preparation has been adapted' (Starr 1982: 132).

Between 1906 and 1980, the FDA consolidated regulatory authority over prescription drugs and gained jurisdiction over all communication from the pharmaceutical industry. Likewise, in the first half of the 20th century, physicians continued to solidify their medical authority over diagnosis of illness and prescribing drugs as treatments (Starr 1982). Both the profession of medicine and the FDA operated to constrain the advertising of pharmaceuticals during most of the 20th century, thereby also constraining consumers' access to pharmaceuticals to treat their aches and troubles. This concurrent consolidation of medical and regulatory authority began to break down in the 1980s.

The emergence of DTCA of prescription drugs: 1981–1996

Direct-to-consumer advertising for prescription medications has fuelled the medicalisation that analysts noted as increasing in Western societies in the 1980s (Conrad 1992). DTCA has become a major source of expanding medical markets and public engagement with medical solutions for life's conditions and problems (Conrad and Leiter 2004).

In 1981, Boots Pharmaceutical (a British firm) issued the first DTC broadcast ad for an ibuprofen product called Rufen and Merck Sharp & Dohme advertised a pneumonia vaccine called Pneumovax (Pines 1999). According to Pines, who was at the FDA at the time, the FDA's first response was shock, and 'Physicians at the FDA generally felt that such advertising was inappropriate' (1999: 492). Yet the very next year, FDA Commissioner Arthur Hull Hayes, Jr. gave a speech before the Pharmaceutical Advertising Council, in which he stated that, 'In sum, my impression is that we may be on the brink of the exponential growth phase of direct-to-consumer promotion of prescription products' (U.S. House of Representatives 1984: 1).

In that speech, Hayes describes the changing dynamics between patients, physicians, and pharmaceutical companies:

There was a time when prescription product advertising to consumers was limited to an occasional institutional ad. Physicians were your industry's sole target audience. Patients had an insignificant voice in choosing prescription products they were given. Generic drugs were not yet an issue. The demographics of consumer publications were such that a very high percentage of the exposures paid for by a prescription product advertiser would be to people who could not possibly use the product. And members of the advertising profession did not want to run the risk of offending physicians by appearing to circumvent them or undercut their freedom of judgment.

It is no longer so. One result of the consumer movement has been increasing numbers of patients who demand a role in the selection of all their health care products. The *Physicians Desk Reference* – as Charlie Baker would be pleased to tell you – is a best seller. It's difficult to remember the last time that the weekly book best seller lists didn't include several volumes about prescription drugs and health care. Specialised health magazines have proliferated. And 90 per cent of prescriptions are now for drugs no one heard of only a generation ago (U.S. House of Representatives 1984: 23–24).

Hayes' speech describes a shift to more consumer-demanded healthcare, with lay persons playing a larger role in determining their own needs and treatments, opening the door to increased medicalisation by health 'consumers'.

In response to this speech, the FDA commissioned a study of physicians and pharmacists regarding patients and prescriptions, and the US House Subcommittee on Oversight and Investigations sent out letters to 37 pharmaceutical companies asking for their position on DTCA (U.S. House of Representatives 1984). Not surprisingly, almost all of the response letters said that the companies would engage in DTCA if their competitors did so. What is striking about the letters is that *they were almost unanimous in their negative responses to the potential of DTCA.* Wayne Davidson, president of the U.S. Pharmaceutical and Nutritional Division of the Bristol-Myers Company, wrote:

> It will be very difficult, if not impossible, for a federal agency (FDA or FTC) to distinguish between when self-diagnosis is possible and when it is not. Where the line is drawn will be the subject of much legal controversy. We are of the opinion it is much better not to attempt to draw the line, but to prohibit this type of advertising to the patient consumer. This type of advertising will also put the prescribing professionals on the defensive in the relationship with their patients, just the reverse of the most productive relationship. . . . (U.S. House of Representatives 1984: 89).

Similarly, Thomas Collins, president of Smith Kline & French Laboratories, replied:

> We do not believe that PDAC [Prescription Drug Advertising to the Consumer] is a good idea. . . . We believe that the chances for damaging doctor-patient relations and for encouraging costly competitive battles are real, while the likelihood that meaningful patient education will occur is small. We certainly welcome, let me stress, the increased consumer participation in health decisions in recent years. It is well for patients to take part, to the extent they wish, in decisions affecting their care. It is however very important to differentiate the capabilities of advertising from those of educational programs. Advertising can inform, but it is not education; and PDAC should not be portrayed as part of the education process (U.S. House of Representatives 1984: 152–3).

Both of these letters voice concerns about consumers' ability to self-diagnose, essentially questioning consumers' medicalisation of their own problems and highlighting the important role that physicians play as gatekeepers in the medicalisation process.

In September of 1982, at the beginning of these explorations, the FDA requested a formal, voluntary moratorium on DTCA (Feather 1998 cited in Pines 1999). In 1983, the FDA issued a policy statement calling for a 'period of cautious restraint on the part of would-be prescription drug advertisers' (50 Fed. Reg. 36677 (1985)). Then in 1985, the FDA withdrew its moratorium, concluding that 'for the time being, current regulations governing prescription drug advertising provide sufficient safeguards to protect consumers' (50 Fed. Reg. 36677 (1985)). According to Pines, the FDA's policy change was 'not intended to open the floodgates for DTC advertising. On the contrary, it was a reluctant recognition by the agency of a new trend, and was intended to ensure that FDA had jurisdiction and that the industry had a framework within which to consider DTC advertising' (1999: 493).

After the FDA withdrew the moratorium, companies increased their print advertising considerably, with companies spending $12 billion in DTCA in 1989 (Medical Advertising News 1999 cited in Pines 1999). However, the cumbersome 'fair balance' and 'brief summary' requirements indirectly kept companies from engaging in DTC broadcast advertising, constraining their outreach to consumers.

DTCA comes to TV: 1997 onward

On 8th, August 1997, the FDA issued draft guidelines for DTCA of product-specific prescription drug broadcast advertisements (62 Fed. Reg. 43171), which described how television and radio ads might fulfill FDA requirements for 'adequate provision' of product information and a 'major statement' of the drug's major risks. Prior to this, these require-ments made TV drug advertising all but impossible.

Under this new interpretation of the regulations, the FDA would allow DTC broadcast advertising if the advertising would provide consumers with the product's approved labelling information through one of four sources: a toll-free telephone number that consumers could call; a concurrent print advertisement containing a brief summary of risk information; a web page (URL) that included the package insert; or additional product information from pharmacists, physicians, or other healthcare providers (Food and Drug Administration 1999). The FDA also announced that it wanted the industry to conduct studies of the effects of DTCA and that it would evaluate the policy in two years (Pines 1999). On 6th, August 1999, the FDA issued its final guidance for DTCA of prescription drugs (64 Fed. Reg. 43197), making very few changes to its original guidelines.

Three types of prescription DTCA would be permitted: product claim advertisements, which included the product name and specific therapeutic claims; reminder advertisements, which gave the name of the drug but did not state its use; and so-called help-seeking advertisements, which told consumers about unspecified treatment possibilities for diseases or conditions (Goldman 2005). From our perspective, all three contribute to medicalisation, with the help-seeking ads the most likely to promote it.

This shift in policy was controversial. Those supporting the change suggested that there would be a public health benefit, depicting broadcast DTCA as 'an excellent way to meet the growing demand for medical information, empowering consumers by educating them about health conditions and possible treatments' (Holmer 1999 quoted in Hollon 2005). Critics voiced reservations, especially regarding how DTCA could lead to overprescribing, how it emphasised newer and more expensive medicines over cheaper existing ones, and regarding 'the medicalising of normal human experience' (Mintzes 2002, Frosch et al. 2007).

Broadcast DTCA has grown enormously in the past years, up from $55 million in 1991 to $4.2 billion in 2005 (USGAO 2006), with 330 per cent growth in DTCA from 1996 to 2005 (Donahue et al. 2007). The ads focus on chronic problems affecting relatively healthy people, with large potential treatment populations and long-term usage, including drugs for allergy, anxiety, obesity, arthritis, erectile dysfunction, and high cholesterol. About 20 prescription drugs make up 60 per cent of the pharmaceutical company spending on DTCA (Hollon 2005) and advertising for one specific drug can have ripple effects for all drugs that are touted for a particular condition. The US Government Accountability Office has estimated that 'each 10% increase in DTC spending within a drug class increases sales in that class by 1%' (2002: 15). DTC ads for drugs to treat erectile dysfunction have become common, especially on television.

DTCA and erectile dysfunction

The Viagra story is by now a familiar one. We need not repeat it in detail here (see Conrad and Leiter 2004, Loe 2004) but will review some points that are relevant to DTCA and medicalisation. In 1992 a consensus conference officially labelled what used to be called impotence as 'erectile dysfunction' and as a biogenic rather than psychogenic problem. In March 1998, the FDA approved Viagra (sildenafil citrate) as a treatment for this condition. In the early days it was marketed primarily to older men with erectile problems and for erectile dysfunction associated with prostate cancer, diabetes, and other medical problems (Loe 2004). Estimates for prevalence ranged from 10 million to half of all American men (Laumann *et al.* 1999). The market potential was not lost on the drug companies, so within a short time Pfizer Pharmaceuticals began advertising Viagra more broadly. With an ageing population, a high prevalence of erectile dysfunction, and an even broader concern with sexual performance, the potential market was huge. DTCA expanded the market to include virtually *any* man who might consider himself as having erectile problems or just wanted a boost in performance (Conrad and Leiter 2004). Within a few years of Viagra's introduction, pharmaceutical competitors came on the scene.

Levitra was introduced in 2003 as a faster drug with fewer adverse effects than Viagra. Levitra ads focused more on recreational uses, targeting 'men who may have successful sexual relationships but simply want to improve the quality or duration of their erections' (Harris 2003). The most visible DTCA spokesman for Levitra was Mike Ditka, a former hardnosed football coach and Hall of Fame player. Levitra became an official sponsor of the National Football League (NFL) and in 2004 became the first pharmaceutical ad during the Super Bowl with its 'Levitra Challenge'. In the week after the Super Bowl, Levitra prescriptions grew by 15 per cent (GSK news release 2004). However, there may be limits to what kind of DTC ads are acceptable for television. The FDA asked Bayer Pharmaceuticals, maker of Levitra, to pull its 15-second spot of 'My Man' ads that promoted Levitra. The ads starred an attractive actress, Marie Silvia – hailed as 'Queen Levitra' by the *Wall Street Journal* – who said how the drug's 'strong and lasting effects' provide a 'quality experience' (Snowbeck 2005). Apparently the ad did not include enough safety information and made a misleading comparison with other drugs for the condition. While the short version of the Queen Levitra ad was pulled, the 45-second version continued to be aired (Snowbeck 2005).

DTCA has shaped and developed the erectile dysfunction drug market. In 2004, drug companies spent over $382 million in advertising these drugs in the US, with sales of $1.36 billion (Snowbeck 2005). The demand for these drugs may have stabilised; doctors wrote 10 per cent fewer new prescriptions in October 2005 than the year before (Berenson 2005). While erectile dysfunction has been firmly medicalised, there may be limits to the demand for medical solutions for sexual difficulties.

From Queen Lydia to Queen Levitra

Lydia Pinkham was the queen of patent medicine. Her product, cooked up in her cellar and composed of herbs and alcohol, epitomises the patent medicine industry in the late 19th and early 20th centuries, which was built largely upon proprietary recipes and grand promises printed on cheap, pulp paper. Patent medicines contributed to a cultural medicalisation of life problems. Advertisements told consumers that they could diagnose their own symptoms and use patent medicines to alleviate those symptoms, without having to resort to consulting physicians. These symptoms ranged from everyday aches and pains, such as being tired or nervous, to serious diseases such as tuberculosis. While over-the-counter medications have continued to fill this self-help niche, during most of the 20th century the profession of medicine and the FDA successfully constrained the advertising of pharmaceuticals to the public, making physicians key gatekeepers to prescription drugs.

Table 1 *Summary of drug advertising activities and implications for medicalisation*

Time periods	Pharmaceutical advertising activities	Implications for medicalisation
Before 1906	Ethical: to physicians Patent: to consumers	Both consumers and physicians are agents of medicalisation
1906–1980	Advertising of prescription drugs to physicians only	Physicians dominate medicalisation
1981–1996	Advertising to physicians; growth in print ads to consumers	Consumers have more information to participate in medicalisation
1997-present	Advertising to physicians; widespread DTCA print and broadcast ads to consumers	Drug industry and consumers become more significant; physicians' centrality decreased

More recently, 'Queen Levitra' was on television, touting Levitra's ability to produce 'strong and lasting effects' and a 'quality experience', alluding to the sexual ability that men may gain (to women's benefit) by taking Levitra. We have come a long way since the days of patent medicine 100 years ago. Yet DTCA hearkens back to those days, in that the pharmaceutical industry is once again reaching out to consumers directly when selling their products and creating wider avenues to the medicalisation of life problems. In this way, the advertising of pharmaceuticals is becoming more like the advertising of over-the-counter medications. In fact, the distinction between prescription drugs and these medications may be less clear now than in the mid-20th century, due to DTCA as well as some pharmaceuticals shifting from prescription to over-the-counter status. For example, Claritin, a well-known antihistamine that was advertised heavily on broadcast media early in the contemporary DTCA era, is now available over the counter.

Pharmaceutical companies' advertising activities have changed considerably, with important implications for medicalisation, as summarised in Table 1. Before 1906, drug manufacturers were split into two increasingly distinct camps: ethical drug manufacturers and patent drug manufacturers. Much of the distinction between these two types of manufacturers was based on the type of advertising that they used to sell their wares: ethical drug companies advertised to physicians only, while patent medicine companies advertised directly to consumers. This gentleman's agreement allowed physicians to legitimise ethical drugs and ethical drug companies to defer to physician's authority in diagnosis and prescribing. During this period, physicians, patent medicine manufacturers, and consumers contributed to expansion of medical definitions and treatments for life problems.

After Congress passed the Food and Drug Act of 1906, the AMA stepped up its efforts to police the boundaries between ethical and patent drug firms, working with the federal government to identify firms that violated the Act. Through this legislation, the government could disrupt the direct relationship between patent drug producers and consumers, protecting consumers in the name of public health. As a result of these efforts, advertising for prescription medications became restricted between 1906–1980 to physicians only and drug companies had a limited role in medicalisation. It is important to note that drug companies always had direct access to consumers for over-the-counter medications. They did not require a medical prescription and were advertised widely. These were typically cold remedies and headache medications, although they would occasionally also encourage medicalisation of new ills such as the 'halitosis' (bad breath) mentioned in Listerine mouthwash advertisements. However, physicians' control over access to pharmaceuticals limited medicalisation.

Around 1981 pharmaceutical companies began to test the gentleman's agreement concerning prescription advertising by initiating limited forays of DTCA. There were no laws against advertising drugs but firms were unsure of what was permissible. A 1985 FDA statement permitted the pharmaceutical industry sufficient latitude to allow a broader engagement with print ads for prescription drugs. The drug companies did not yet venture into broadcast ads due to the difficulty of fulfilling the FDA's requirements regarding the 'major statement' of risks and side effects of drugs.

The reinterpretation of FDA advertising guidelines in 1997 had major implications for DTCA, especially on television. Now drug companies could market directly to consumers. Physicians became gatekeepers for drugs advertised direct to consumers rather than initiators of pharmaceutical treatments: 'Ask your doctor if [name of drug] is right for you'. The drug industry and consumers, facilitated by DTCA, have become major players in medicalisation with physicians relegated to somewhat less of a role (Conrad 2007). In fact, direct access to consumers has increased the pharmaceutical industry's incentive to medicalise human problems, encouraging consumers to self-diagnose and request drugs that they see on TV. Furthermore, the Internet has become another direct avenue from pharmaceutical companies to consumers, and one that is not limited to national boundaries. This electronic form of DTCA can already be considered as a factor in internationalising medicalisation. Some Internet sites bypass physicians altogether with a veneer of medical oversight.

The impacts of DTCA on medicalisation and health are complicated. DTCA can raise awareness about disease and risk, and provide some useful medical information for consumers, although most physicians believe that DTCA does not provide balanced information (Perri *et al.* 1999, Hollon 2005). DTCA has significant impact on patient demands, physicians prescribing, and by implication, medicalisation. DTC advertising leads to increased requests for advertised medicines and more prescriptions (Mintzes *et al.* 2003). A study by Kravitz *et al.* (2005) sent trained standardised patients to physicians. The 'patients' presented symptoms of either major depression or adjustment disorder and made DTC-related requests of a brand specific drug, a general class of drugs, or no request. 'Patients' who made brand-specific requests or general requests for drugs were much more likely than patients who made no requests for drugs to receive a prescription. Requesting medications increased the amount of prescribing, at least for these two disorders. What is disturbing here is that although there are no data to support the use of antidepressants for adjustment disorder, half of those who requested it, based on DTCA, received prescriptions. The authors conclude that DTCA 'may stimulate prescribing of more questionable than clear indications' (Kravitz *et al.* 2005: 2000).

The scrutiny and criticism of DTCA appears to be increasing from various quarters. U.S. Senate Majority Leader Bill Frist (a physician) expressed concerns that DTCA creates a wedge between physicians and patients (Henderson 2005). An article in *Advertising Age* questioned whether recent drug safety scares may shift the balance of power back to physicians (Thomaselli 2005) as consumers respond to cases such as Vioxx's well-advertised entry and quick removal from the market. In July 2005, the drug industry drafted guidelines that called for a period of notifying doctors about new drugs before advertising to consumers (Saul 2005a). These new voluntary guidelines would 'virtually eliminate 15-second spots' because they do not provide enough time to list risks, and require that all ads will be submitted to the FDA for review before they are used (Saul 2005b). While it is too early to judge the impact of these changes on medicalisation, it seems doubtful that these changes would significantly decrease the roles of DTC advertising and consumers on medicalisation.

Conclusion

While DTCA appears to be flourishing, even FDA personnel seem concerned about its effects on medicalisation. In a meeting about DTCA, Janet Woodcock, the director of the FDA's Center for Drug Evaluation and Research, highlighted two concerns: 'First, that many common and relatively minor complaints of daily life represent diseases. This has been called the medicalisation of life. And second, the perception that all life complaints can and perhaps should be treated with a pill' (Food and Drug Administration 2003: 22). Broadcast DTCA is now only permitted in the US and New Zealand and is prohibited in the United Kingdom and most developed countries. Should DTC advertising be introduced in Europe (Watson 2003), most of the same issues would exist (Metzl 2007).

One of the ironies of DTCA is that it expands the relationship of drug companies, physicians and consumers, returning it to a situation similar to Lydia Pinkham's day, when the drug manufacturers had a direct and independent relationship with consumers. It encourages self-diagnosis and requests for treatment. It allows pharmaceutical companies to create specific markets for their products and promote them to waiting customers. Of course, with stronger government regulation and a more powerful medical profession, the situation is also different from what it was a century ago. The extravagant claims of Lydia Pinkham's day are constrained by laws, but modern advertising is both more subtle and sophisticated than what was available to the patent medicine peddlers. It seems clear that the pharmaceutical industry and consumers are becoming increasingly important players in medicalisation and that DTCA facilitates this shift.

References

Anderson, A. (2000) *Snake Oil, Hustlers and Hambones: the American Medical Show*. Jefferson: McFarland and Company.

Applegate, E. (1998) *Personalities and Products: a Historical Perspective on Advertising in America.* Westport, CT: Greenwood Press.

Berenson, A. (2005) Sales of impotence drugs fall, defying expectations, *New York Times*, December 4, 1, (http://www.nytimes.com/2005/12/04/business/yourmoney/04impotence.html?ex=1178596800&en=9a037a1bdd97025e&ei=5070) (accessed May 5, 2007).

Conrad, P. (1992) Medicalization and Social Control, *Annual Review of Sociology*, 18, 209–32.

Conrad, P. (2005) The shifting engines of medicalisation, *Journal of Health and Social Behavior*, 46, 1, 3–14.

Conrad, P. (2007) *The Medicalisation of Society: On the Transformation of Human Conditions into Treatable Disorders*. Baltimore: Johns Hopkins University Press.

Conrad, P. and Leiter, V. (2004) Medicalisation, markets and consumers, *Journal of Health and Social Behavior*, 45, Extra Issue, 158–76.

Conrad, P. and Schneider, J.W. (1992) *Deviance and Medicalisation: From Badness to Sickness*. Philadelphia: Temple University Press.

Crossen, C. (2004) Fraudulent claims led U.S. to take on drug makers in 1900s, *Wall Street Journal*, Oct. 6, B1.

Donahue, J.M., Cevasco, M. and Rosenthal, M.B. (2007) A decade of direct-to-consumer advertising of prescription drugs, *New England Journal of Medicine*, 357, 673–81.

Feather, K.R. (1998) Presentation before the Institute for International Research, Washington, D.C., Sept. 14, 1998.

Food and Drug Administration. (1999) *Guidance for Industry: Consumer-Directed Broadcast Advertisements Questions and Answers*. (http://www.fda.gov/cder/guidance/1804q&a.htm) (accessed May 16, 2007).

Food and Drug Administration. (2003) *Direct-to-Consumer Promotion: Public Meeting, September 22 and 23, 2003.* (http://www.fda.gov/cder/ddmac/DTCmeeting2003.html) (accessed July 7, 2005).

Freidson, E. (1970) *The Profession of Medicine.* New York: Dodd, Mead.

Frosch, D.L., Krueger, P.M., Hornik, R.C., Cronholm, P.F. and Barg, F.K. (2007) Creating demand for prescription drugs: a content analysis of television direct-to-consumer advertising, *Annals of Family Medicine*, 5, 1, 6–13.

Goldman, M. (2005) Direct-to-consumer advertising: benefit to patients? Drug and Marketing Publications (http://www.drugandmarket.com/default.asp? section=feature&article=042205)

GSK news release. (2004) GlaxoSmithKline news release, (http://www.gsk.com/media/archive. htm#nolink) (accessed May 15, 2007).

Harris, G. (2003) Levitra, a rival with ribald ads, gains on Viagra, *New York Times*, September 18, C5.

Harrison-Barbet, A. (1994) *Thomas Holloway: Victorian Philanthropist: a Biographical Essay.* Egham: Royal Holloway, University of London.

Henderson, D. (2005) With advertising under siege, drug makers rethink their marketing message, *The Boston Globe*, July 31, E1.

Hollon, M.F. (2005) Direct-to-consumer advertising: a haphazard approach to health promotion, *JAMA*, 293, 16, 2030–3.

Holmer, A.F. (1999) Direct-to-consumer prescription drug advertising builds bridges between patient and physician, *JAMA*, 281, 4, 380–4.

Israel, F.L., (ed.) (1968) *1897 and 1908 Sears Roebuck Catalog.* New York: Chelsea House Publishers.

Kravitz, R.L., Epstein, R.M., Feldman, M.D., Franz, C.E., Azari, A., Wilkes, M.S., Hinton, L. and Franks, P. (2005) Influence of patients' requests for direct-to-consumer advertised antidepressants: A randomised controlled trial, *JAMA*, 293, 16, 1995–2002.

Laumann, E.O., Paik, A. and Rosen, R.C. (1999) Sexual dysfunction in the United States: prevalence and predictors, *JAMA*, 281, 6, 537–44.

Loe, M. (2004) *The Rise of Viagra.* New York: New York University Press.

Medical Advertising News. (1999) Chart, 20.

Metzl, J.M. (2007) If direct-to-consumer advertisements come to Europe: lessons from the USA. *Lancet* 369: 704–06.

Mintzes, B. (2002) Direct to consumer advertising is medicalising normal human experience, *British Medical Journal*, 324, 908–11.

Mintzes, B., Barer, M.L., Kravitz, R.L., Bassett, K., Lexchin, J., Kazanjian, A., Evans, R.G., Pan, R. and Marion, S.A. (2003) How does direct-to-consumer advertising (DTCA) affect prescribing? A survey in primary care environments with and without legal DTCA, *Canadian Medical Association Journal*, 169, 5, 405–12.

Perri, M., Shinde, S. and Banavali, R. (1999) The past, present and future of direct-to-consumer drug advertising, *Clinical Therapy*, 21, 10, 1798–811.

Pines, W.L. (1999) A history and perspective on direct-to-consumer promotion, *Food and Drug Law Journal*, 54, 489–518.

Pinkus, R.L. (2002) From Lydia Pinkham to Bob Dole: what the changing face of direct-to-consumer drug advertising reveals about the profession of medicine, *Kennedy Institute of Ethics Journal*, 12, 141–58.

Saul, S. (2005a) Drug industry proposes limits on advertising, *The New York Times*, July 22, C4.

Saul, S. (2005b) Drug makers to police consumer campaigns, *The New York Times*, August 3, C7.

Shorter, E. (1992) *From Paralysis to Fatigue: A History of Psychosomatic Illness in the Modern Era.* New York: Free Press.

Simmons, J.G. (2002) *Doctors and Discoveries: Lives That Created What Medicine is Today.* Boston: Houghton Mifflin.

Snowbeck, C. (2005) FDA tells Levitra to cool it with ad, *Pittsburgh Globe-Gazette*, April 19. (http://www.post-gazette.com/pg/05109/490334.stm) (accessed May 14, 2007).

Spillane, J.F. (2004) The road to the Harrison Narcotics Act: drugs and their control, 1875–1918. In Erlen, J. and Spillane, J.F., (eds) *Federal Drug Control: The Evolution of Policy and Practice*, New York: Pharmaceutical Products Press.

Starr, P. (1982) *The Transformation of American Medicine*, New York: Basic Books.

Thomaselli, R. (2005) PR seems to be the Rx to get around DTC rules: firms confirm pharma is seeking ways to live with (but not skirt) guidelines, *Advertising Age*, 26 September, 6.

U.S. Government Accountability Office. (2002) *Prescription Drugs: FDA Oversight of Direct-to-Consumer Advertising has Limitations*. Washington, D.C.: U.S. General Accountability Office.

U.S. Government Accountability Office. (2006) *Prescription Drugs: Improvements Needed in FDA's Oversight of Direct-to-Consumer Advertising*. Washington, D.C.: U.S. Government Accountability Office.

U.S. House of Representatives. (1984) *Prescription Drug Advertising to Consumers. Staff Report Prepared for the Use of the Subcommittee on Oversight and Investigations of the Committee on Energy and Commerce, House of Representatives*. Washington, D.C.: U.S. Government Printing Office.

Watson, R. (2003) EU health ministers reject proposal for limited direct to consumer advertising. *BMJ*, 326, 1284.

Wertz, R. and Wertz, D. (1989) *Lying In: a History of Childbirth in America*. New Haven: Yale University Press.

Young, J.H. (1961) *The Toadstool Millionaires: a History of Patent Medicines in America Before Federal Regulation*. Princeton, N.J.: Princeton University Press.

3

Waking up to sleepiness: Modafinil, the media and the pharmaceuticalisation of everyday/night life

Simon J. Williams, Clive Seale, Sharon Boden, Pam Lowe and Deborah Lynn Steinberg

Introduction

Recent years have witnessed an upsurge of sociological interest in pharmaceuticals, including on-going research on the regulation of the pharmaceutical industry (Abraham 1995, Abraham and Lewis 2002); related debates on globalisation and the pharmaceutical industry (Busfield 2003); the role of the pharmaceutical industry in so-called 'disease mongering' (Blech 2006) and the medicalisation of society (Conrad 2007); the meaning and use of medications in lay culture and everyday life (Britten 1996, Gabe and Lipshitz-Phillips 1982); and studies of pharmacies, pharmacists, prescribing and concordance (Britten *et al.* 2004, Stevenson *et al.* 2002, Harding and Taylor 1997).

Pharmaceuticals and the media
Another key issue concerns the role and function of the media in relation to pharmaceuticals and the 'pharmaceuticalisation' of everyday life. Media coverage of pharmaceuticals, as previous studies have shown, is complex and variable over time. Often, when drugs are first discovered or licensed, media coverage tends to be positive in tone and content, including enthusiastic headlines extolling the virtues of a new 'breakthrough' or 'wonder drug'. Nelkin (1995), for example, highlights the wave of enthusiastic media attention which Prozac (dubbed the 'feel good drug') received in the 1990s, with Viagra subsequently following in its footsteps. *If* or *when* unwelcome side effects become apparent, however, or misuse of some sort on the part of doctors or the lay populace is detected, then negative constructions or demonisation of the drug in question seems to predominate or prevail. We see this very clearly, for example, with regard to media coverage of benzodiazepines over time. Gabe and Bury (1996), for instance, note the considerable media attention devoted to the risks of taking benzodiazepines over the last 40 years. When first prescribed to patients in the 1960s, the media gave these drugs a 'generally enthusiastic welcome' (1996: 76). As this new generation of tranquillizers became more popular, however, their therapeutic value ceased to be 'newsworthy', with more critical coverage developing from the 1970s onwards – coverage highlighting both the risks of the drugs' 'addictive potential' and journalistic imperatives for 'dramatisation' and 'personalisation' (1996: 78; see also Cohen 1983).

Media treatment of medicines and drugs then, as Seale comments, 'demonstrates a tendency to idealise or stigmatise, creating oppositional extremes' (2002: 152; see also Entwistle and Sheldon 1999). Rarely do the media present a 'balanced picture of harm and benefit contained in a single substance' (2002: 148). Whilst the actions of drug companies indeed are often subject to criticism, the media are frequently accused of promoting rather than challenging pharmaceutical interests, wittingly or unwittingly: a point which returns us to notions of 'disease mongering' mentioned above (see, for example, Blech 2006 and Moynihan *et al.* 2002). Whilst 'new' media such as the Internet, moreover, may provide spaces or forums to challenge or resist these processes, they may equally provide new avenues or channels for the medicalisation or pharmaceuticalisation of daily life (see, for example, Fox *et al.* 2005).

Modafinil: the shape of things to come?
It is against this backdrop of recent sociological work on pharmaceuticals in general and the role of the media in relation to pharmaceuticals in particular, that this chapter is located. Our focus, in contrast to the previous studies mentioned, is on British newspaper coverage of the new wakefulness-promoting drug Modafinil, a drug manufactured by the American Pennsylvania-based pharmaceutical company, Cephalon, under the brand name Provigil[1]. Originally approved for the treatment of excessive daytime sleepiness associated with narcolepsy, Provigil has now received both Food and Drugs Administration (FDA) and Medicines and Healthcare products Regulatory Agency (MHRA) approval for the treatment of excessive sleepiness associated with obstructive sleep apnoea. Additionally, it has now received approval for the treatment of excessive sleepiness associated with 'shift work sleep disorder' (www.Cephalon.com; www.provigil.com). It is also used 'off label' for a variety of other sleepiness- and fatigue-related conditions. Modafinil, it is claimed, is a drug that truly breaks new ground. Unlike former stimulants, Modafinil is an *eugeroic* drug (Greek for 'good arousal') that can promote alert wakefulness with none of the buzz, jitteriness or highs and lows of its predecessors. It has also been found to improve memory, cognitive performance, mood and concentration – *i.e.* a nootropic or 'smart' drug with demonstrable cognitive 'enhancing' effects (Turner 2003, Hart 2006). Perhaps most remarkably of all, Modafinil does not disturb sleep and only seems to promote wakefulness 'under conditions where vigilance is sought by the person who has taken it' (Wolpe 2002: 391).

The market potential of this drug is huge, as Cephalon's year-on-year sales figures clearly attest (http://www.Cephalon.com). Cephalon, indeed, appear to be a very enterprising company having joined the list of companies included in the Fortune 1000 annual rankings of America's largest corporations (http://www.Cephalon.com). A recent feature on Cephalon in *Business Week* – tellingly entitled 'Eyes wide open' and proudly posted on Cephalon's own website – suggests that the Company business strategy can serve as a model or exemplar for other biopharmaceutical enterprises. 'Cephalon's scientists', the article proclaims, 'respond to doctors who report that Provigil is helpful with various disorders such as sleep apnoea. Collaborating with doctors, Cephalon can provide the FDA with persuasive data on these ailments, and thus expand the use of the drug' (http://www.Cephalon.com).

The potential market for Modafinil, however, extends far beyond the boundaries or confines of the doctor's surgery or sleep clinic, including a significant 'lifestyle' market. As with a range of other so-called 'enhancement' technologies designed to make us 'better than well' or 'better humans' (Miller and Wilsdon 2006; Parens 1998), if not 'better than human', Modafinil therefore raise some intriguing if not disturbing social and ethical questions, which in this particular case translate into debates over the prospects and possibilities of a world in which wakefulness, for better or worse, can be more or less readily conjured at will or medicated/manufactured on demand.

What then do the media make of Modafinil? How is Modafinil being constructed and represented in the British press? What cultural commonsenses are being circulated and conveyed regarding this new drug? Are there any particular points of convergence or consensus, contestation or controversy in this newspaper coverage? And what does this tell us about the role of the media in the medicalisation or pharmaceuticalisation of alertness and the governance of sleepy bodies in contemporary culture? These are some of the questions this chapter seeks to address. Before doing so, however, a word or two about methods.

Methodological matters: retrieving and analysing newspaper stories

This chapter is part of a broader project on social constructions of sleep in the British print news media. The study, in this respect, was primarily concerned with news print media constructions of sleep, rather than audience reception of and responses to these messages, or the institutional arrangements involved in the production of news. Articles for the study were retrieved from the Lexis Nexis archival database. Our selection of six UK national newspaper texts (*Times, Guardian, Independent, Daily Mail, Daily Mirror, Sun* and their Sunday equivalents) was influenced by knowledge of the circulation figures and readership profiles (obtained from circulation figures on the Newspaper Marketing Agency website www.nmauk.co.uk), alongside sampling for contrasting tone, format and political orientation.

All searches started from the date of first loading onto the Lexis Nexis database until 31st August 2006[2], using search terms such as 'Modafinil', 'Provigil', 'wakefulness promoting drugs'. As it was major press coverage we were most interested in, for the purposes of this particular chapter at least, articles were selected from inclusion in the study if any of these search terms were mentioned three or more times. This resulted in a total of 54 articles across all papers sampled, with a higher proportion of articles in the (former) 'broadsheet' or more 'serious' papers – a finding which held across all search criteria deployed.

A variety of different techniques are now available for the analysis of media materials in general and newspapers in particular, including more quantitative forms of analysis such as content analysis and more qualitative forms of analysis such as discourse analysis (Fenton *et al.* 1998, Potter 1996). Given our particular interest in the meanings and messages conveyed in this press coverage, our own approach favoured a more qualitative or interpretive analysis. Articles were read, catalogued and compared in terms of key words and phrases, key developing issues and storylines, the use of 'experts' and/or research data, evidence of medicalisation/disease mongering, how the reader was addressed/drawn into the piece, and the vocabulary used, particularly the 'moral' messages, rhetorical styles and/or emotional overtones of these selected articles. These emerging themes and issues were then used as an aid to further qualitative, interpretive analysis on how such articles constructed their subject matter and how they were intended to be read. Although primarily qualitative in nature, however, our analysis also included some basic frequency counts regarding this press coverage as background and context for the more in-depth qualitative analysis of themes and storylines that follow.

Discourses and debates: medicalisation and beyond

Four main themes emerged in our sample, which pertain respectively to the following uses and abuses of Modafinil/Provigil: (i) clinical treatment of medical conditions; (ii) lifestyle choices; (iii) military operations; (iv) (un)fair competition. The distribution of these four themes according to newspaper and year are shown in Tables 1 and 2 respectively.

As Table 1 indicates, the most commonly reported theme in our sample as a whole pertained to (un)fair competition, primarily in the field of sport, followed by medical matters, lifestyle choices and finally military 'uses' and 'abuses' of the drug. The *Times* was the paper in which the clinical and medical applications of Modafinil featured most often, followed by the *Mail* and the *Independent*. Concerns over the drug as a lifestyle choice were also most evident in the *Times*, followed by the *Independent* and the *Mail*. Military coverage, in contrast, was almost exclusively featured in the *Guardian*, centred on an issue which materialised in 2004 – see Table 2. Similarly, most of the press coverage of sporting

Table 1 *Press coverage of key themes by newspaper**

Paper/Theme	Times	Guardian	Independent	Mirror	Mail	Sun	(sub) Total
Medical	7		3		6	1	17
Lifestyle	5		2		2		9
Military		4			1		5
Competition	10	11	6	3	2	1	33
(sub) Total	22	15	11	3	11	2	64

Table 2 *Press coverage of key themes by year**

Year/Theme	'98	'99	2000	'01	'02	'03	'04	'05	'06	(sub) Total
Medical	2				1	2	6	4	2	17
Lifestyle							4	3	2	9
Military						5				5
Competition						25	7	1		33
(sub) Total	2				1	27	22	8	4	64

* Figures in both Tables 1 & 2 exceed the total article count (54) given that two or more themes may appear in any one article.

competition across all newspapers pertained to an event that materialised in 2003 and rumbled on into 2004 – see Table 2.

As Table 2 indicates, apart from a couple of early stories surrounding the clinical launch of the drug in 1998, most press coverage has occurred since 2003, with sport (as noted above) featuring prominently in 2003, and a more even distribution of themes the following year, 2004. Since then, however, medical and lifestyles themes seem to have predominated, though our sample, to repeat, only takes us up to the 31st of August 2006.

It is to a more detailed account of each of these key themes that we now turn.

Medical conditions: from narcolepsy to . . . ?

The earliest reportage of Modafinil in our newspaper sample occurred in 1998, when the drug was first launched in the UK. A story in *The Independent* (4 March 1998), for example, entitled 'Wonder wake-up pill boosts alertness' (in the 'News' section of the paper), informs us that 'A wake-up pill that increases alertness and boosts memory in people who are sleep deprived was launched yesterday'. The drug, it is noted, 'could provide the *pharmacological equivalent of the electric light bulb*' (our emphasis). The bulk of the story, however, rests content with mere reportage, with no comment or judgement passed, of the somewhat delimited claims and ambitions of the manufacturers of the drug. The medical director of Cephalon UK, Dr Colin Makland, for instance, is quoted as saying that there are 'no plans' to explore the drug's potential as an 'alertness pill'. 'All our activities', Makland assures us, 'have been in the area of narcolepsy. If we wanted to seek another indication for the drug we would have to go back and conduct other studies'.

Much of the newspaper coverage of the medical use of Modafinil, as this suggests, has narcolepsy somewhere in the storyline. This however took a variety of forms, from straight-forward matter-of-fact reportage about the efficacy of the drug in the treatment of narcolepsy

– sometimes written by doctors or sleep experts themselves, particularly in the (former) 'broadsheet' or more 'serious' papers – to more glowing reports of how this new 'wonder' drug transforms lives through personal stories and case studies drawn from sufferers of narcolepsy themselves. We see this, for example, very clearly in an article in the *Times* (27 July 2004), in its 'Features' section, which opens as follows:

As a teenager, Brendan Maguire had to be careful not to laugh. If he did, he could fall to the floor in a deep sleep. He spent most of his days in bed because he always felt sleepy.

Maguire has narcolepsy and his life was transformed two years ago by a new drug, Provigil, that allows him to live an almost normal life. 'Now I can do a 12 hour shift' at a call centre', he says.

The *Independent* (28 September 2000), in similar fashion, carried a story (in the 'Features' section of the paper) entitled 'Health: the fast asleep club'. 'For sufferers from narcolepsy', the paper notes, 'fighting weariness is a way of life. They live everyday as if the previous 48 hours have been sleepless'. Sufferers are then drawn into the storyline, such as Kerry James, (a college lecturer), who became so bad that she 'frequently fell asleep during meetings, over meals and once even had to find an empty teaching room in which to take a nap on the floor'. Kerry, the reader is told, was eventually diagnosed with narcolepsy and since then she has been taking Provigil, which means she 'can now go virtually through the day without needing to nap'.

Gradually however, over time, these narcolepsy-based storylines are joined if not eclipsed by newspaper coverage of other clinical or experimental applications of the drug, again largely uncritical in tone and content, for conditions such as obstructive sleep apnoea (OSA), multiple sclerosis, 'shift work sleep disorder' (SWSD) and Attention Deficit/Hyperactivity Disorder (ADHD). The *Times* (15 August 2005), for example, in an article by a medical doctor, informs readers that Modafinil is useful not simply for the treatment of narcolepsy but also for '. . . treating the daytime sleepiness associated with obstructive sleep apnoea'. Readers are also told in this article that '*The New England Journal of Medicine* has recently reported on another use for Provigil: 10 per cent of night-shift workers find that the irregular hours makes them excessive sleepy while they are working'. The 'careful double-blind trial', carried out by the Division of Sleep Medicine at Harvard University and researchers from other centres, the doctor informs the reader, 'showed that Provigil did bring about modest improvement in the night-shift workers' problems: they were more alert when working and their accident rate on the way home was significantly reduced' (*Times*, 15 August 2005).

Further justifications for these new clinical uses of Modafinil could also be discerned in other stories, particularly in terms of accident reduction or prevention. Another doctor, for example, in his 'Drug of the Week' column (Sunday Surgery, Health Section) in the *News of the World* (11 April 2004), asks his readers:

Do you nod off during the day? *It's a serious problem if you're operating machinery or driving.*

Readers are then informed that:

Provigil (also known by its generic name Modafinil) boosts alertness and is prescribed in severe cases such as people with Parkinson's disease. *Many of Britain's four million night workers could use it too* (our emphases).

Sleep experts and doctors are then drawn upon to provide further endorsement for these particular uses of the drug. The use of doctors and sleep experts indeed was a common theme in our newspaper sample. The *Daily Mail*, for example, quotes a consultant neurologist who stresses how this drug 'really can transform people's lives', adding that it 'should help people with a *wide range of conditions* where fatigue is an issue. *The potential benefits are enormous*' (14 September 2004, our emphasis).

As for the merits of Modafinil in relation to ADHD, another article in the *Daily Mail* a year later (20 December 2005) – this time with the attention-grabbing headline 'Anti-sleep drug can calm down little Barts' – opens in the following fashion:

> Research shows that Provigil can have a dramatic effect on behaviour and attention span in children with Attention Deficit Hyperactivity Disorder (ADHD).

The article, however, in a variant on the theme of medical expertise, concludes with a quote from a representative of the ADHD information service, Andrea Bilbow, who states that: 'the "stay awake" pill had already been tested on adults with ADHD and seemed to work well . . . If it proves to have few side-effects, then it is obviously going to be a useful treatment'.[3]

Beyond this condition's specific coverage, however, it was possible to discern other more amorphous, nebuluous, references made in the press to notions of 'excessive' sleepiness or an 'inability to stay awake' as the clinical target or referent for this drug. The *Daily Mail* (14 September 2004), for example, informs its readers that 'doctors say Provigil (also known as Modafinil) – now licensed for use in the UK for the treatment of *excessive sleepiness* – is *great news for patients plagued by the inability to stay awake*'. Provigil, the reader is told, repeating the medical mantra, 'can change people's lives. Patients who have been living in *a fog of sleepiness* for years find that in a few days the clock has been turned back and they're able to live a normal life again' (our emphases).

There is then, as these extracts clearly show, precious little in this newspaper coverage that is critical or even cautious of this expanding list of clinical conditions for which Modafinil is currently prescribed or potentially applicable. Instead, the guiding template seems to be a matter-of-fact or upbeat style of reportage about the clinical benefits of this drug, aided and abetted by personal testimonies, the latest findings from clinical trials and/or the views of this or that sleep expert. At most what one gets here in the way of critical coverage are occasional qualified comments such as 'Provigil has revolutionised the treatment of narcolepsy *but* cannot be used indiscriminately. It may cause over-excitement or irritability' (*Times*, 8 September 2003) or a lone, dissenting if not 'maverick' voice, cast in these very terms, such as John Mortimer, whose polemical piece in the *Daily Mail*, (14 November 2002) is comically entitled: 'A pill to help my memory? Forget it!' Modafinil, he notes:

> . . . a drug once used for sleeping sickness (sic), can – so Professor Robins of Cambridge University has discovered – sharpen short-term memory and help problem-solving and planning.

But forgetfulness, Mortimer protests, can be 'a great excuse' or 'alibi'. 'How terrible it would be', then, 'if the usual excuse of forgetting met with: "Well take a large dose of Modafinil and come back when you've remembered"'. And suppose, 'in a moment of weakness, that we took the medicine?', he continues:

> How painful, how unbearably overcrowded our minds would become . . . So let us keep the clouds of unknowing where we can hide the past, lit by only occasional shafts of memory.

Whilst Mortimer provides something of a lone or dissenting voice as far as the clinical merits of Modafinil are concerned, he is nevertheless in good company when it comes to media concerns over the use of this drug for non-clinical reasons or non-medical purposes.

Lifestyle choices: flexible workers and party people
Another key concern articulated and conveyed in this press coverage of Modafinil pertains to the potential of the drug to further blur the boundaries between the aforementioned 'legitimate' treatment of medical conditions and its 'uses' and 'abuses' as a (lifestyle) drug of choice.

Again we see this articulated in the press in a variety of ways. The *Daily Mail* (5 January 2004), for example, in a brief article on the drug, notes how 'critics fear this could lead to the use of Provigil being extended to healthy people who are simply short of sleep'. 'Patients with demanding careers and lifestyles', the reader is told, are 'already beginning to ask for Provigil'. The *Times*, in a spate of articles in 2004 and 2005, articulates and amplifies similar concerns. The *Sunday Times* (4 July 2004), for instance, carried a story – in the 'Home News' section of the paper – proclaiming in the headline that 'Downtime is over as pill offers 24-hour living'. 'A pill that helps users feel wide awake after long periods without sleep', it states, 'is being tipped as *the latest lifestyle "wonder drug" to hit Britain*' (our emphasis). The article then proceeds to use the situation in America to raise concerns in the UK:

> . . . the pill has been credited with fuelling the rise of the '24-hour society' by helping truckers, students, night-clubbers and international travellers stay awake through the night or cope with jet lag. The drug has achieved sales of £250m a year.

> Now the same thing may happen here. The Medicines and Healthcare products Regulatory Agency has quietly decided to loosen the tight restrictions governing who can be prescribed Provigil.

American users, the reader is told, 'describe in enthusiastic terms how the pill has enabled them to stay awake without the jitteriness and anxiety brought about by large doses of caffeine'. As such, it is claimed, the drug could 'undergo the "Viagra phenomenon", in which its main use would be to *enhance lifestyles rather than treat medical conditions*' (our emphasis).

Various expert viewpoints are then drawn into the picture, this time sounding a strong note of caution and concern about the potential uptake of this drug. The director of the centre for cognitive neuroscience at the University of Pennsylvania, for example, is quoted as saying that Provigil had already accelerated America's trend towards becoming a 24–7 society and would do the same in Europe. 'This drug enables us to be even more worka-holic and obsessed with accomplishments and productivity', she says, 'It takes away the natural checks on that tendency – like needing to go to bed' (*Sunday Times*, 4 July 2004).

This particular article is also notable for the way in which it draws the manufacturers of Modafinil, Cephalon Inc. into the storyline. On the one hand, it is noted, how: 'Cephalon, the company behind Provigil, says it is horrified at the lifestyle "abuse" of its drug'. On the other hand, readers are informed that:

> Cephalon's earlier marketing told a different story. Two years ago it was reprimanded by the Food and Drugs Administration – America's regulatory body – for the 'dissemination of false or misleading promotional materials for Provigil' (*Sunday Times*, 4 July 2004).

Two further stories in the *Times* underline these concerns. In the first, which appeared in the 'Features' section of the paper (27 July 2004), it is noted how, in the US, Provigil is 'largely used for non-medical reasons – to sustain a party or business lifestyle without apparent penalties'. Provigil, the article continues: '. . . *blurs the line between treating a medical condition and a lifestyle choice*' (our emphasis), noting moreover, through a direct quote from an eminent British sleep scientist, that 'we don't know the long-term effects of using drugs to stay awake longer'. 'What we do know', the sleep scientist stresses, 'is that there are powerful mechanisms for sleep and no natural ways to override them, so it's a potentially dangerous thing to do'.

The second article, a year later (2 July 2005), in the 'Features: Body & Soul' section of the newspaper, provides something of a curtain raiser for a *Times*-sponsored event at the Science Museum's Dana Centre entitled 'Night Creatures'. The key question this article poses is whether or not we 'really want to stay up all night?'. Increasingly, the article notes, 'especially in America, people are resorting to the new "stay-awake" drug Provigil, which promises six or seven hours of alertness with no problems falling asleep afterwards'. 'But is this the right way to deal with the issue?' the article asks:

> Drawing an analogy with food, are we indulging in a form of '*somorexia*', a deluded and unhealthy belief that we can do without sleep . . . Or is the whole notion that our 24/7 lifestyle is creating a nationwide sleep-debt itself a delusion?

The problem, the article concedes, in somewhat pessimistic tones, is that:

> . . . there is little chance of turning back the clock on our open-all-night society. We have expanding demands on our time and increasing numbers of people do shift work. Hence the attraction of Provigil, a drug originally licensed to treat narcolepsy . . . Its sales have rocketed in the past two years, from $300 million to $600 million (£166 to £322 million).

A further variant on this type of coverage concerned a more specific focus on Internet access to this drug. The *Independent* (18 April 2006), for example, in a Features section article entitled 'My pills.co.uk', ran a story alerting readers to the fact that 'some of the world's best selling prescription drugs are not simply being taken by the sick but are also being used as "lifestyle medications"' though the Internet. The ease of availability of virtually every kind of drug over the Internet, readers are told, has meant that 'many people are now simply *bypassing their doctor* and *self-prescribing* medicines which they hope will improve their looks, job performance or prowess in the bedroom rather than treat a specific condition or disease' (our emphases). There is even, the article warns, a 'darker side to the "lifestyle drugs" industry', in which 'many drugs sold online are fakes that at best will not have the effect and at worst could kill'. Provigil is then drawn into the picture, alongside other drugs such as Prozac, Ritalin, Viagra and the statin Lipitor, noting how strict regulations on prescribing Provigil were eased two years ago, and how 'clubbers are using it to keep partying through the night, while businessmen are buying it to help them through long days in the office, and students are taking it to keep revising'. Doctors, it adds, have 'warned that the drug can be psychologically addictive and can induce headaches and nausea'.

Not all articles, however, appeared to share these concerns, or at the very least seemed happy to endorse more widespread usage of the drug beyond any immediate clinical concerns. An article in the *Times* (15 August 2005), for example, entitled 'The pill that's a wake up call' (again by a medical doctor in the 'Features' section of the paper), proclaimed in unqualified fashion, that:

Judges who fall asleep on the bench, Cabinet ministers who can't keep awake at public functions, and MPs who nod off in front of the television cameras in the House of Commons would all present a more alert and intelligent face to the world, and the cameras, if they took a small dose of Provigil (Modafinil) before their appearance.

But 'most importantly', the article goes on to state:

> ... lives would be saved on the roads, especially motorways, if long-distance drivers, whether in giant trucks or Minis, not only had regular rests but took the occasional Provigil tablet when there was any danger of them dropping off.

Modafinil then, as this press coverage suggests, is indeed construed and constructed as a somewhat 'controversial' drug, precisely because of its appeal to a wide range of potential 'users' and 'abusers' in the name of work or play, productivity or pleasure. There is, however, another potential market for the drug that looms large in this press coverage, one that takes us far beyond the realms of civil society.

Military operations: sleep as a 'commodity' of war
Military uses or deployments of Provigil also featured in our newspaper sample, particularly in the (former) 'broadsheets' or more 'serious' papers. As with medical uses of the drug, some of this coverage adopted a rather matter-of-fact style of reporting, often in the context of a broader discussion of the drug and its potential applications. An article in the *Daily Mail* (5 January 2004), for example, informs its readers of a 'study of military helicopter pilots' which 'showed that the drug helped them stay alert and remain capable of performing complex tasks for almost two days without sleep', without passing any significant comment.

Other stories, however, chose instead to frame Provigil in terms of broader coverage of the problems of sleep deprivation for the military and the various efforts, both actual and on the horizon, to combat it. The *Guardian* (29 July 2004), for example, in an article entitled 'Wired awake: soldiers in the field go for days without rest', notes how dealing with sleep deprivation is a 'perennial problem for the military', before drawing upon various military experts in the field to comment on this problem. 'While drugs to combat sleepiness have their risks', Greg Belensky – from the Walter Reed Army Institute of Research in Silver Spring, Maryland – states, 'so too does deploying troops who aren't sufficiently rested'. Belensky's team, the reader is told, has 'studied the effects of caffeine, speed and Provigil . . . on troops kept awake for up to 85 hours'. Readers are also informed of other cutting edge developments, such as research conducted at the University of Wisconsin, Madison, funded by the US Department of Defence, which hopes, through investigation of the 'biological secrets' that allow migrating birds to exist on little or no sleep, to develop 'not simply stimulants that keep you awake, but drugs that go a long way to *removing* the need for sleep' (our emphasis). Efforts are also underway at Belensky's lab, the reader is told, to:

> ... *turn sleep into a commodity of war, much like bullets and fuel.* In the next few months, troops will go on exercises wearing wristwatches that carefully monitor how much sleep they get . . . The wristwatches will also give advice on what stimulants, if any, should be taken, depending on the mission ahead. 'The idea is to *turn sleep into an item of logistic supply*', says Belensky. 'We want to *treat it like fuel – how much do people have, how long will it last them, and when do we need to fill them up again*', he says (our emphases).

In this way, then, a variety of scenarios are rehearsed which provide, in effect, speculations on the future of sleep not simply for the military but for us all as these developments catch hold, take off or spill over into society at large.

Particular flashpoints could also be discerned in this coverage. Perhaps the most striking illustration of this occurred in a spate of further *Guardian* articles in July 2004, couched in something of an investigative style designed to shock the reader. A headline on the first page of the *Guardian* (29 July), for example, read: 'Provigil is a drug able to keep pilots and combat troops awake for days. Now the *Guardian* can reveal the MoD bought thousands of pills in advance of the Iraq war'. The MoD, the article reports:

> . . . admitted to buying more than 24,000 Provigil pills, which are licensed in Britain only to help people with rare sleeping disorders shrug off daytime sleepiness. Experts say the new drug could be used 'off licence' to keep pilots and special forces troops awake on little sleep.

'Military interest in Provigil', the reader is told, 'is fuelled by a desire to find alternatives to existing stimulants used to keep troops awake', noting how 'The US military has stepped up research into Provigil since the 1990s'.

Continuing this line of investigative journalism, another article in the paper the following day (30 July 2004), by the same reporter in the 'Home pages' section, reveals that scientists at Qinteg, the MoD's main research contractor, are 'preparing to publish research into the potential military uses of Provigil' with the results due to be discussed in detail in October at the European Sleep Research Society meeting in Prague. 'Yesterday', the article continues, (presumably in response to the previous day's story), 'the MoD said that the armed forces were not issued or prescribed Provigil or any other stimulants for operation or training purposes, adding that military stocks of Provigil were used only to treat those with narcolepsy and other rare sleep disorders'. The article concludes, however, by noting how 'military forces around the world have been investigating Provigil as a means of keeping fatigued troops sharp in combat, since the early 90s', including recommendations by French military researchers on the use of Provigil for missions lasting 24 hours without sleep. A short letter in the 'Comment & Analysis' section of the paper duly follows, bearing the contentious title 'Letters: General's claim adds insult to injury'. In it Vice Admiral Ian Jenkins (Surgeon General, Ministry of Defence), reiterates that: 'The MoD does not use Provigil for performance-enhancing purposes'.

What we see here, then, in this newspaper coverage of Modafinil and the military, are a range of both real and imagined future scenarios which enable the press once again to rehearse a series of developments and debates, concerns and anxieties about the 'uses' and 'abuses' of this drug, both on and off the battlefield. This includes the 'leaky' or 'hybrid' matter of the soldier's body itself, which is increasingly being reworked or reconfigured through a series of cyborg couplings or human-machine fusions (*cf.* Haraway 1990, Gray 1995), thereby turning sleep into a 'commodity of war' – see also Ben-Ari (2003) on this theme.

(Un)Fair competition? The race to get ahead

The fourth and final theme in our sample, widely reported upon across all newspapers, concerned the use of Modafinil in sport. Much of this coverage centred on the controversial case of the US 100 and 200 metres sprinter Kelli White, whose use of Modafinil proved to be the first test case of its kind for the International Association of Athletics Federation (IAAF). This indeed was the only story covered by all the newspapers in our sample.

We see this unfolding drama, for example, very clearly in a spate of articles in the *Times*, in 2003, which report how White tested positive for Modafinil at the 2003 World Championships in Paris, and how controversy followed, not simply over the reason for White's use of this drug (a self-proclaimed case of narcolepsy) but whether or not Modafinil was in fact, or should be, classified as a 'banned substance' for IAAF purposes. In one article, for instance, bearing the header 'White's second positive test serves only to muddy the waters' (*Times*, 13 November 2003, 'Sport' section), we are told that:

> Within a fortnight of the World Championships, Robert Wagner, White's agent, handed a 25-page statement to Lunquist [chairman of the IAAF medical commission] which argued that Modafinil could not be considered a banned substance. Later that month, Cephalon, the worldwide manufacturer of the drug, sent a submission to Dick Pound, chief executive of WADA [World Anti-Doping Authority]. Paul Blake, senior vice-president of Cephalon, argued that Modafinil was not a stimulant, but a 'wake-promoter' and could not be related to any stimulant on the list. 'It is a separate pharmacological entity', Blake said.

A subsequent article in the *Guardian* (19 May 2005), however, cast in more confessional tones, reveals how White, in coming clean to the World Anti-Doping Agency (WADA) at a hearing in Montreal, experimented with a 'cocktail of banned substances':

> 'I was offered a lot of things and asked to test them to see if I responded better to certain products', she said. 'I was like a guinea pig. I tried a lot of stimulants and Modafinil suited me perfectly. The same for tetrahydrogestrinone (THG), which helped put on muscle very quickly'.

As for White's claim to be suffering from narcolepsy, this, the reader is informed, was simply a 'cover story': ' "I never suffered from narcolepsy", White said. "I never even knew the word existed until a few hours after the announcement of my positive test" '.

Whilst White is singled out for sustained press attention here, coverage also extended to reports of other athletes implicated in this controversy. The *Sun* (1 January 2004), for example, ran a story entitled 'Track ace Kelli fails test No. 2' in which it is reported that 'Now the US Olympic Committee have revealed White is one of seven athletes who failed drugs tests last summer'. 'All seven athletes', the *Sun* notes, 'are challenging the results. If Modafinil use is proved, it results in disqualification at the event at which a positive test occurred – but no suspension'.

Modafinil, then, may very well be regarded as the latest in a long list of drugs and substances banned for use in sport, raising once again the spectre of unfair advantage. It is nonetheless, as White's particular story clearly attests, instructive on a number of further counts, not least in terms of: (i) bogus appeals to medical conditions as (il)legitimate grounds for using this drug; (ii) the ensuing IAAF and WADA deliberations as to whether or not Modafinil was in fact a 'banned substance', and; (iii) the role of the pharmaceutical industry itself in this critical test case. In reporting on these issues, therefore, the press again provide an effective vehicle for the articulation of a broader series of moral concerns and agendas regarding the potential uses and abuses of this drug in the competition or race to get ahead.

Discussion and concluding remarks

This study has been primarily concerned with the social construction of Provigil/Modafinil in the British national press. Further work, as such, is clearly needed not simply in terms of the social construction of this drug in other types of media, both new and old, but in relation to questions of audience reception/response as well as the specific cultures and institutional arrangements involved in the production of 'newsworthy' stories in this domain. Our data nonetheless, returning to the questions posed at the beginning of this chapter, are instructive on a number of counts and at a number of different levels.

In terms of the content of newspaper coverage, constructions of Modafinil in the British press, as we have seen, cluster around four key themes pertaining to the medical, lifestyle, military and sporting uses and abuses of the drug – with greatest coverage accorded to the latter theme (see Table 1), due to a particular scandal emerging in 2003 concerning the use of the drug (see Table 2). Whilst medical uses of Provigil, in this respect, are largely portrayed in unproblematic, uncritical terms – proclaiming it something of a 'wonder drug' for the treatment of a growing range of medical conditions – other non-medical uses are a source of considerable press concern, if not outright condemnation, particularly as a lifestyle drug of choice or as performance enhancer. The concern here seems to be the manner in which Modafinil, like Viagra before it, serves to further blur the lines between treatment and enhancement (itself of course a socially constructed and contested distinction): the latest expression indeed of on-going social, ethical and legal debates in relation to a variety of new medical technologies (Rose 2007, Miller and Wilsdon 2006, Brown and Webster 2004, Parens 1998). Military deployments of Modafinil also receive critical coverage, though tempered somewhat by an acknowledgement that sleep deprivation is a real problem in certain (sustained) military operations, and that whilst drugs to combat sleep(iness) have their risks, so too do sleepy soldiers in combat. To the extent, moreover, that reportage of these military deployments provides an opportunity for the press to rehearse a series of current concerns and future scenarios regarding the fate or changing fortunes of sleep in so-called '24/7 society' (Moore-Ede 1993), it serves to further draw the reader into the story line turning sleep into a matter of public concern. The press, as such, are active constructors and arbitrators in these debates, thereby helping raise both the profile of this new drug and the problem of sleep(iness) in the public's mind.

So what then does this tell us about the relationship between medicine, the media and the pharmaceutical industry? Certainly the 'textual link' between people in society has never been more evident; everything these days, it seems, is mediated in one way or another by the media, though not all mediation is 'textual' of course. But does this, as Kroll-Smith (2003) implies in his musings on the social construction of sleepiness in the media, provide an opportunity to critique the more pedestrian or prosaic versions of the medicalisation thesis in terms of medicine's attempts to capture public problems? Is what we are seeing here, in other words, a more or less clear-cut case of 'Direct-to-Patient' medicalisation on the part of the media, bypassing the doctor in the process? Well, yes and no. Certainly the news has become a key way, if not *the* key way, of mediating a pharmaceutical to the public, particularly in countries such as Britain where DTCA is not permitted. To the extent, furthermore, that what is conveyed is 'news', it is likely to be treated more seriously or credibly by readers than a full-page glossy ad in a magazine for this or that Big Pharma product[4]. To the extent, however, that journalists regularly draw on sleep experts and doctors of various sorts as sources of authority and expertise, and to the extent that the traditional doctor-patient relationship itself is sometimes used as a media template or framing device for these stories – including calls for patients to visit their doctor if they are 'excessively sleepy' or suffering from particular sleep 'problems' or 'pathologies' – then the degree to which these media constructions can truly be regarded as 'extra institutional' forms of 'rhetorical authority' and/or bypassing the doctor is open to question. At most, it seems, the traditional doctor-patient relationship and the institutional authority of medicine is being 'reworked' or 'reconfigured' rather than replaced or bypassed altogether in and through this newspaper coverage. The media, in short, may play a variety of roles in relation to both doctors and drugs.

This press coverage of Provigil, however, also alerts us to the *limits of a solely or strictly medicalised interpretation of these issues*, at least as far as the media are concerned. To the extent, indeed, that press concerns about the potential uptake of this drug cluster around or centre on its actual or potential non-medical uses and abuses, then what we see here is the articulation or amplification of a series of cultural anxieties about the *pharmaceuticalisation* rather than the medicalisation of alertness, sleepiness and everyday/night life. Pharmaceuticalisation, in this sense, refers to the transformation of human conditions, capacities or capabilities into pharmaceutical matters of treatment or enhancement. As such it overlaps with but extends far beyond the realms of the medical or the medicalised, and serves further to blur the boundaries between treatment and enhancement. In praising and/or criticising these developments, however, the media may (inadvertently) contribute to them, diffusing information and raising awareness of pharmaceutical products in the public's mind, thereby facilitating their potential uptake in everyday/night life. Media coverage of pharmaceuticals then, as this suggests, may have paradoxical, or at the very least unintended, consequences.

Here we arrive at the final question posed at the beginning of this chapter as to what all this tells us about the (bio)politics of alertness and the governance of sleepy bodies in contemporary culture? Why precisely would society want to regulate or govern sleepiness and alertness in this way? Who benefits? Again, of course, this is a question which takes us far beyond the realms of the strictly medical or the medicalised to broader questions about the role of pharmaceuticals in society. One evocative or provocative answer to these questions comes in the shape of Agger's (2004, 1989) musings on 'Fast Capitalism'[5]. Capitalism, Agger argues, has appreciably *speeded up* since Marx's time, and even since the post World War II period – see also Gleick (2000) and Virilio (1986) on this theme. The key words here are *'acceleration'* and *'instantaneity'*. The rate of 'communicating, writing, connecting, shopping, browsing, surfing, and working has increased', Agger (2004: 3) proclaims, particularly since the advent of communication technologies and the Internet. Boundaries of all sorts, as a consequence, have become blurred or broken down. 'Nothing today', it seems, is 'off limits to the culture industries and other industries that colonize not only our waking hours but also our dreaming' (2004: 3). The adjective *fast*, in this sense, is intended to modify our sense of capitalism in two main ways: first, through the compression of time (*cf.* Harvey 1989 and Giddens 1991) as the 'pace of everyday life quickens in order to meet certain economic imperatives and to achieve control'; secondly, through the 'erosion of boundaries, which are *effaced by a social order bent on denying people private space and time'* (Agger 2004: 3–4, our emphasis).

Nothing, to repeat, is off limits in the 24/7 era of *fast* capitalism. Sleep or sleepiness, as such, becomes a 'problem', or at least a potential problem, in need of a solution in an increasingly time-hungry, incessant culture: a quick fix technical solution, in the case of Modafinil, which amounts to a further colonisation of the body and everyday/night life through pharmacological means. To the extent, moreover, that sleep represents an attempt to 'slow down' (*cf.* Honoré 2004) or 'opt out' of society, albeit temporarily or periodically – *cf.* Schwartz's (1970) notion of sleep as a 'periodic remission' from society – then our 'ways of escape' are effectively closing down or diminishing in the 24/7 era of 'fast' capitalism where achievement is prized, alertness is emphasized and vigilance is valorised. Modafinil, indeed, is simply the first of a new wave of drugs, including CX717 currently on trial, that provide the pharmacological means to prolong, promote and police our wakefulness, fuelling claims (rightly or wrongly) that sooner or later we will be able to pharmacologically or genetically 'switch' or 'turn sleep off' altogether (Lawton 2006: 34).

These issues in turn raise related questions of 'pharmacological Calvinism' (Conrad 2007, Healy 1997, Klerman 1972): the Puritan, disciplined, ascetic belief, that is to say, that we need to work hard in order to achieve a valued goal or objective rather than take drugs or medications as a short-cut to success. To the extent that drugs such as Modafinil *embody* the Protestant work ethic (*cf.* Weber 1930), or at the very least display an 'elective affinity' to it – providing us with the pharmacological *means* to remain alert, sharpen concentration, boost cognitive performance and work even harder at the things we value – then the very notion of pharmaceutical Calvinism takes on potentially troubling new dimensions[6]. Expressed more broadly, what this amounts to perhaps is yet another prime expression or glimpse of our (future) 'neurochemical selves' (Rose 2002) and of the intimate or inextricable links now forged between what Rose (2007) appositely terms 'somatic ethics' (*i.e.* ethics that accord a central place to corporeal, bodily existence) and the 'spirit of biocapital'; developments that carry profound implications for who we are and who we want to be.

In *reporting* on these developments and *rehearsing* these dilemmas and debates, the press, in effect, are not simply alerting us to the pharmacological fortunes of this new drug, but providing us with a potent preview or portent of what may one day, for better or worse, through biotechnological tampering or tinkering of various kinds, become a society in which sleep is rendered *optional* if not (entirely) *obsolete*: A 'utopian' or 'dystopian' future, depending on your point of view, but one which potentially implicates us all given our current status as sleeping as well as waking beings.

Notes

1   The terms Modafinil and Provigil will be used interchangeably throughout the chapter and reflect, in large part, their usage in the British newspaper sources surveyed.

2   Dates of first loading for newspapers on the LN database were as follows: *The Guardian* 1984, *The Times* 1985, *The Independent* 1988, *The Mail* 1992, *The Mirror* 1995, *The Sun* 2000.

3   Cephalon's supplemental New Drug Application (sNDA) to market Modafinil (under the brand name Sparlon) for the treatment of ADHD in children and adolescents was rejected by the FDA in August 2006.

4   Thanks to one of the anonymous referees for drawing this point to our attention.

5   Thanks to one of the anonymous referees for highlighting this source.

6   At the time of writing, the *Times Higher Education Supplement* has just published a full-page feature on the use of Modafinil and other so-called 'smart drugs' in academia: a growing trend in the global academic community, it is suggested, in a time squeezed, performance pressured, results-driven culture such as ours (Tysome 2007; see also Bee 2007 and Martin 2007). This in turn suggests that concerns over the 'uses' and 'abuses' of Modafinil in relation to wakefulness are now joined by, if not eclipsed by, concerns over its cognitive/brain-boosting qualities as a 'smart drug', particularly in educational contexts but also more widely in society at large.

References

Abraham, J. (1995) *Science, Politics and the Pharmaceutical Industry: Controversy and Bias in Drug Regulation*. London: UCL Press.

Abraham, J. and Lewis, G. (2002) Citizenship, medical expertise and the regulatory state in Europe, *Sociology*, 36, 1, 67–88.

Agger, B. (1989) *Fast Capitalism: a Critical Theory of Significance*. Urbana: Illinois Press.

Agger, B. (2004) *Speeding up Fast Capitalism*. London: Paradigm Publishers.

Bee, P. (2007) Smart drugs for straight As, *Timesonline*, 14 May. http://www.timesonline.co.uk

Ben-Ari, E. (2003) Sleep and night time combat in contemporary armed forces: technology, knowledge and the enhancement of the soldier's body. In Steger, B. and Brunt, L. (eds) *Night-time and Sleep in Asia and the West: Exploring the Dark Side of Life*. London: Routledge Curzon.

Blech, J. (2006) *Inventing Disease and Pushing Pills*. London: Routledge.

Britten, N. (1996) Lay views of drugs and medicines: orthodox and unorthodox accounts. In Williams S.J. and Calnan, M. (eds) *Modern Medicine: Lay Perspectives and Experiences*. London: UCL Press.

Britten, N., Stevenson, F., Gafaranga, J., Barry, C. and Bradley, C. (2004) The expression of aversion to medicines in general practice consultations, *Social Science and Medicine*, 59, 1495–503.

Brown, N. and Webster, A. (2004) *New Medical Technologies and Society: Reordering Life*. Cambridge: Polity Press.

Busfield, J. (2003) Globalization and the pharmaceutical industry revisited, *International Journal of Health Services*, 33, 3, 581–603.

Cohen, S. (1983) Current attitudes towards benzodiazepines: trial by the media, *Journal of Psychoactive Drugs*, 15, 109–13.

Conrad, P. (2007) *The Medicalisation of Society*. Baltimore: Johns Hopkins University Press.

Entwhistle, V. and Sheldon, T. (1999) The picture of health? Media coverage of the health service. In Franklin, B. (ed.) *Social Policy, the Media and Misrepresentation*. London: Routledge.

Fenton, N., Bryman, A. and Deacon, D. (1998) *Mediating Social Science*. London: Sage.

Fox, N.J., Ward, K.J. and O'Rourk, A.J. (2005) The 'Expert Patient': empowerment or medical dominance? *Social Science and Medicine*, 60, 6, 1299–309.

Gabe, J. and Bury, M. (1996) Risking tranquilliser use: cultural and lay dimensions. In Williams, S.J. and Calnan, M. (eds) *Modern Medicine: Lay Perspectives and Experiences*. London: UCL Press.

Gabe, J. and Lipshitz-Phillips, S. (1982) Evil necessity? The meaning of benzodiazepine use for women patients from one general practice, *Sociology of Health and Illness*, 4, 2, 201–9.

Giddens, A. (1991) *Modernity and Self-identity*. Cambridge: Polity Press.

Gleick, J. (2000) *Faster: the Acceleration of Just About Everything*. London: Abacus.

Gray, C.H. (1995) *The Cyborg Handbook*. London: Routledge.

Gray, C.H. (2002) *Cyborg Citzen*. London: Routledge.

Haraway, D. (1990) *Simians, Cyborgs and Women*. London: Free Association Press.

Harding, G. and Taylor, K. (1997) Responding to change: the case of community pharmacy in Britain, *Sociology of Health and Illness*, 19, 5, 547–60.

Hart, C. (2006) Modafinil attenuates disruptions in cognitive performance during simulated night-shift work, *Neuropsychopharmacology*, 31, 7, 1526–36.

Harvey, D. (1989) *The Conditions of Postmodernity*. Oxford: Blackwell.

Healy, D. (1997) *The Antidepressant Era*. Cambridge: Harvard University Press.

Honoré, C. (2004) *In Praise of Slowness: how a World Wide Movement is Challenging the Cult of Speed*. London: Orion Books.

Klernman, G. (1972) Psychotropic hedonism vs. pharmacological Calvinsm, *Hastings Centre Report*, 2, 4, 1–3.

Kroll-Smith, S. (2003) Popular media and 'excessive daytime sleepiness': a study of rhetorical authority in medical sociology. *Sociology of Health and Illness*, 25, 6, 625–43.

Lawton, G. (2006) Get up and go, *New Scientist*, 18 February, 34–8.

Martin, N. (2007) Intelligence drugs could be as 'common as coffee', *Telegraph* online 19 April. http://www.telegraph.co.uk

Moore-Ede, (1993) *The 24/7 Society: the Risks, Costs and Consequences of a World that Never Stops*. London: Piatkus.

Moynihan, R., Health, I. and Henry, D. (2002) Selling sickness: the pharmaceutical industry and disease mongering, *British Medical Journal*, 324, 13 April, 886–91.

Miller, P. and Wilsdon, J. (eds) (2006) *Better Humans? The Politics of Human Enhancement and Life Extension*. London: Demos.

Nelkin, D. (1995) *Selling Science: how the Press Covers Science and Technology*. New York: W.H. Freeman.

Parens, E. (ed.) (1998) *Enhancing Human Traits: Social and Ethical Implications*. Washington D.C.: Georgetown University Press.

Potter, J. (1996) *Representing Reality: Discourse, Rhetoric and Social Construction*. London: Sage.

Rose, N. (2002) Neurochemical selves, *Society*, 41, 1, 46–59.

Rose, N. (2007) *The Politics of Life Itself: Biomedicine, Power and Subjectivity in the Twenty-First Century*. Princeton, N.J.: Princeton University Press.

Schwartz, B. (1970) Notes on the sociology of sleep, *Sociological Quarterly*, 11, 485–99.

Seale, C. (2002) *Media and Health*. London: Sage.

Stevenson, F., Britten, N., Barry, C., Bradley, C. and Barber, N. (2002) Perceptions of legitimacy: the influence on medicine taking and prescribing, *Health* 6, 1, 85–104.

Turner, D. (2003) Cognitive enhancing effects of Modafinil in healthy volunteers, *Psychopharmacology*, 165, 3, 260–9.

Tysome, T. (2007) Pills provide brain boost for academics, *Times Higher Education Supplement*, 29 June, 6–7.

Virilio, P. (1986) *Speed and Politics: an Essay on Dromology*, Transl. Polizotti, M. New York: Semiotext(e).

Weber, M. (1930) *The Protestant Ethic and the Spirit of Capitalism*. London: Allen and Unwin.

Wolpe, P.R. (2002) Treatment, enhancement, and the ethics of neurotherapies, *Brain and Cognition*, 50, 387–95.

4

Pharma in the bedroom . . . and the kitchen. . . . The pharmaceuticalisation of daily life

Nick J. Fox and Katie J. Ward

Introduction

The home computer and Internet have provided a window for the pharmaceutical industry into people's domestic spaces, both for information about and purchase of pharmaceuticals via burgeoning online pharmacies (Fox *et al.* 2005c, 2005d). In the US, where direct-to-consumer (DTC) marketing of pharmaceuticals is permitted, lifestyle products such as Viagra have been a test-bed for more general conditions including allergies, insomnia and acid reflux, and 'lifestyle marketing' of products is a major element of product promotion (Applbaum 2006: 446). In 2005, the drugs with the biggest marketing budgets were a sleep aid, a heartburn drug, two cholesterol-lowering pharmaceuticals and an asthma drug (Med Ad News staff 2006), while the total DTC spend was $4.2 billion, rising by 20 per cent per year since 1997, twice as fast as marketing to physicians, which stood at $7 billion per year in 2005 (General Accountability Office 2006). Pfizer's motto on its corporate website: *Life is our life's work*, suggests that the world's largest pharmaceutical company acknowledges the significance of this orientation.

In this chapter we will examine in greater detail some of the consequences of this new emphasis on lifestyle in the production, marketing and consumption of pharmaceuticals. While much of the chapter is discursive, integrating a range of literatures from the social sciences, economics and business, and health services research, we will illustrate our themes by drawing upon data from a study of pharmaceutical consumption (Fox *et al.* 2005a, 2005b, Fox and Ward 2006).[1] This study looked at how particular pharmaceutical products were consumed, from medical applications to usage based on lifestyle choices. Thus orlistat (Xenical) and similar preparations designed to aid weight loss among obese patients, are sometimes used to manage diet or even to sustain low body weight, while the erectile dysfunction (ED) drug sildenafil (Viagra) has been used by both men and women recreationally to enhance sexual performance (Fox and Ward 2006). In both their medical and non-medical applications, these pharmaceuticals are associated with intimate personal aspirations concerning sexual fulfilment, attractiveness and body shape, and affecting particular aspects of normal daily life.

We shall argue that people's homes are increasingly the places where drug companies make their money from these highly profitable and popular drugs. These are often available only by prescription, yet are marketed formally or informally to consumers as well as health professionals (Applbaum 2006, Moynihan *et al.* 2002). Such products mark a step-change in the *domestication* of pharmaceuticals from a previous generation's medicine cabinet of over-the-counter analgesics and antacids. Linked with the emergence of Internet pharmacies and online consultations, and the emphasis by pharmaceutical corporations upon lifestyle, we will also suggest that we are seeing the *pharmaceuticalisation* of domestic life. By this, we mean that alongside other areas of domestic space, the bedroom and the kitchen are now foci for pharmaceutical marketing and consumption, incorporating citizens and the pharmaceutical industry into a network of social relations that extends from the personal to the corporate arenas.

'Lifestyle' and pharmaceuticals

The emergence of a range of pharmaceuticals in the 1990s that focused less on curing disease and more on enhancing people's quality of life led social scientists to attend to the characteristics of these drugs. Lexchin (2001: 1449) suggested two categories of 'lifestyle drugs': those intended or used for a purpose that 'falls into the border zone between the medical and social definitions of health' (for example, male hair loss or compromised sexual potency), and those that 'treat diseases that derive from a person's lifestyle choices' (for example, obesity or nicotine addiction). Flower (2004: 182) was more wide-ranging, arguing that some lifestyle drugs are intended to 'satisfy a non-health-related goal or [treat] problems that lie at the margins of health and well being'. His categorisation of lifestyle drugs includes 'herbal' and 'alternative' remedies, street drugs, and those such as alcohol and caffeine that occur naturally in consumer products but are rarely used clinically. He then defined two kinds of lifestyle drugs: those specifically designed and manufactured to serve a lifestyle purpose (for example, sildenafil [Viagra], orlistat [Xenical] and methadone), and those designed for one clinical use but with a secondary lifestyle use (for example, the anti-hypertensive minoxidil and finasteride, an anti-androgenic drug used to treat prostatic hypertrophy, both of which can be used to address androgenic alopecia). To these we may add a further category: drugs marketed and prescribed for a non-lifestyle use, but also used by consumers for different, lifestyle purposes. For example, the drug norethisterone, usually prescribed as a contraceptive, hormone replacement therapy or to prevent menorrhagia, was increasingly requested by women in order to delay menstruation during holidays or other events, making it a lifestyle drug when used in this way (Shakespeare *et al.* 2000). Fox and Ward (2006) found a similar transgressive use of weight loss pharmaceuticals among anorexics and sildenafil among young men and women.

In many ways, these efforts at definition have been superseded by events. As noted earlier, the advent of the Internet and marketing to consumers has led to burgeoning emphasis on the lifestyle-related qualities of drugs from cholesterol-lowering preparations to anti-allergenics (Applbaum 2006). Writing in 2008, what is perhaps of more interest is the impact of this emphasis on people's lives in an era when there is a pill for every ill, but perhaps more significantly, an ill for every pill (Mintzes 2002: 909). To this end, we turn first to the processes whereby pharmaceutical consumption has been domesticated.

The domestication of pharmaceutical consumption

During the last century, the home became the focus for many technological advances that transformed the private lives of citizens and domestic social relations (Cockburn 1994, Ormrod 1994). Studies have examined the impact of technology on home life, while other theorists have recognised that the translation of technology into the domestic arena is contingent on existing social relations. Thus, for example, Ormrod (1994) points to the conservative views of gender relations that surrounded the innovation of the microwave oven. Marketers appealed both to female concerns with cooking for the family and male interests in technology to sell their product (1994: 56). The domestication of computing shows how inventors of this technology failed to foresee the uses in a domestic setting and the subsequent shaping of the technology for uses such as games (Haddon 1994: 85) and, more recently, convergence of computers with digital media. These examples suggest that translation of a technology such as medical chemotherapy to a domestic setting is not straightforward.

Our research on consumer experiences and attitudes to pharmaceutical use provides insights into the domestication of pharmaceutical consumption. This research was part of a larger study on consumption of pharmaceuticals and the role of the Internet (Fox *et al.* 2005a, 2005b, Fox and Ward 2006) that used online ethnographic methods in order to access hard-to-reach groups of pharmaceutical consumers (some of whom used these drugs without medical supervision). This entailed observation and participation in Internet discussion forums and subsequent interviews with participants, typically by e-mail. Our studies examined the use of sildenafil (Viagra) and related drugs such as tadalafil (Cialis) to achieve or enhance male sexual potency, and orlistat (Xenical or Alli) and phentermine (Adipex or 'phen') as adjuncts to weight loss. These serve as exemplars of the emergence of products that are consumed on a continuum from a medicalised and professionalised context through to a privatised context located in the bedrooms, kitchens and sitting rooms of users. We undertook research in a number of online message forums devoted to the use of these pharmaceuticals, over a period of months during 2003. The Xenical groups were preponderantly female, while the Viagra group was mixed; no information on ages was gathered. In each forum, KJW subscribed as a member and announced her identity as a researcher. After a period of acculturation to the norms of the values of the groups, she participated actively in the forums, asking questions of participants. Some responded to the questions via the forum, while others chose to e-mail their responses privately, which provided the opportunity for a total of 36 follow-up e-mail interviews. The forums and names of participants have been changed throughout to protect anonymity, and postings have been reproduced verbatim.[2]

We found three aspects to the domestication of pharmaceutical consumption. The first concerns how lifestyle prescription drugs are acquired. Our research found that this was increasingly by online consultation via a home computer rather than from a GP surgery or hospital clinic. Online pharmacies cater to a global market for health-care products (Fox *et al.* 2005c), and some of the best-selling pharmaceutical products have been developed with such markets in mind. In the UK, 'e-clinics' use online consultations to assess people's suitability for medications such as sildenafil and orlistat, before selling these products directly to consumers. One respondent told us that the Internet was his preferred medium for obtaining sildenafil:

> I buy my viagra via the Internet, and I have had no concerns. It's fast, easy and cheaper than the local pharmacy. I used to search the Internet for all sorts of information regarding [erectile dysfunction], but I decided I needed to get on with my life and stop obsessing about this problem (Robert).

Surfing the net can be the route to opportunistic self-medication, as in this example:

> I just happened to buy a sample pack of generic Cialis online to try it. I was very interested in its ability to not be affected by food – or not as much by food, as my online friend from Australia has revealed (Mike).

Similarly, for those seeking pharmaceuticals to help them lose weight, the Internet can be more 'user-friendly' than a doctor's office. For Daisy, the Internet was a way to avoid the inconvenience of a doctor's appointment, but perhaps more importantly, the risk of not getting the medication:

> My doctor wanted to put me on Xenical and it was so expensive and I have no insurance so [the Internet] was cheaper and I didn't have to listen to my doctor, because I have a thyroid problem and they think I should just eat right and exercise (which works) but I

have no patience so I went with buying online. When I was on the Phen I saw a cheesy doctor who prescribed it to anyone . . . but the drive and the office visit monthly was costly so I just thought I would try online.

Even where people obtained Xenical from their doctor, much of the day-to-day experience of using the drug took place in a domestic context, through contacts with a range of support networks provided by the manufacturer. One participant on the Xenical discussion board mentioned this support:

Did you know that Xenical offers a free support program to those that have been prescribed [Xenical]? They have a dietician that you can call via 1-800 and they also have a welcome package which includes a video, an information binder, food guide, and a 20 day meal planner. The dietician supports you for 3–6 months via postal service, email, internet site, and phone. They are very good. The support you get from them, your physician and this site is everything you need.

The second way in which lifestyle drugs domesticate the experience of pharmaceutical consumption derives from the personal and often private nature of the conditions for which these drugs are designed, treating 'embarrassing' conditions such as impotence, hair loss, obesity and so forth. Commenting on the personal impact of impotence, a respondent suggested that 'one never realises how good it feels to be "hard" when . . . unable to achieve that state of being'. Jane contacted the Viagra discussion group to ask for help with her boyfriend's impotence:

I don't have a clue what to believe and what not to believe. I looked up ED and this is what it said: Erectile dysfunction, or ED, can be a total inability to achieve erection, an inconsistent ability to do so, or a tendency to sustain only brief erections. I would say my boyfriend has the last of these . . . He's already had Viagra and we both enjoyed the results, immensely, but he's not willing to go to a doctor to get it. Can anybody help me sort this all out, please?

Obesity was for many of our respondents a condition that impacted on their daily lives:

I am getting married this August, and I won't even let my fiancé see me naked, I won't make love naked, and when it's hot as heck outside, I won't sleep nude! And I don't like that, I want to feel more comfy in my skin, or lack of it (Mary).

Gemma had told only a limited number of people about her use of Xenical and perceived a stigma attached to taking the drug, which she connected to her negative stereotypes of overweight people as slothful, bad mannered and greedy: she perceived use of Xenical as 'a sign of personal weakness that I couldn't do this on my own'. Sarah felt she was a victim of discrimination by a slim society within which she was an 'intruder':

I want to be able to go into a shop and not worry about if I can fit any of their clothes. I want to swim. I want to achieve a goal. . . . There are so many disadvantages to being overweight, people find you unattractive, clothing, sickness, limiting in experiences, uncomfortable-ness.

Thirdly, lifestyle drugs domesticate the consumption of pharmaceuticals because they are aimed at activities that are related to domestic life. For those within stable relationships, sexual activity tends to take place within private-home spaces, while weight-loss drugs such as Xenical are intended as adjuncts to a diet that limits fat intake, and so is directly associated with the food preparation that takes place in people's kitchens and the monitoring of weight loss in bathrooms and bedrooms. John used the terminology of a scientific experiment to describe his and his wife's intimate encounters using pharmaceuticals:

> I for one am very excited and impressed, and we are trying as a husband and wife to discount or not let the 'placebo effect' influence our experience with Cialis. I don't feel that I have extreme ED, but sometimes I am amazed at how 'dead' my part can be . . . so to have anything work well – and as well as Cialis, I am ready and willing to use it.

For those using weight loss drugs, the pills must be part of a carefully planned diet, especially as excess fat intake can lead to diarrhoea. For Ellen, this meant a new emphasis on cooking and food preparation:

> I don't follow Weight watchers or the Xenical pack or anything else for that matter. I have done so in the past, and I find that the recording of everything that I eat, or following what someone else designs for me to eat, doesn't work for me. I'm really trying to do the lifestyle change this time, so I'm really trying to change how I cook and what I put into the food I cook, and making the new way the normal way.

One respondent made links between two domestic activities: sexual encounters between husband and wife, and the management of food intake (sildenafil works best on an empty stomach):

> I am just tired of having to plan our times together, and on an empty stomach as I watch my wife eat dinner or a meal. But being able to plan and be successful together is a small price to pay I guess. The alternative – not having Viagra to use – would obviously be worse. And, then I just eat afterwards (Mike).

It has been said that when a new technology emerges, the first profitable exploitation in a public arena is for sexual purposes, as was the case for both the video cassette and the Internet (Perdue 2002: 1, Rheingold 1995: 102). Perhaps then, it is unsurprising that Viagra has been among the first pharmaceutical technologies to be exploited in a non-medical setting, and has been a cash cow for Internet pharmacies. Since we conducted our research in 2003, these outlets have become mainstream and now retail very many compounds, although still with a strong emphasis on 'lifestyle' conditions. In this section we have identified three elements that underpin the domestication of pharmaceutical consumption, in the sense of re-locating consumption within the home. However, it is worth noting that these processes may also reflect the other sense of 'domestication': rendering safe something wild or unpredictable.[3] While pharmaceuticals are potent and potentially toxic chemicals, the removal of consumption from the doctor's surgery to the computer in the back bedroom may domesticate pharmaceuticals symbolically as well as practically. This is of relevance as we now turn to the broader cultural, economic and political aspects of pharmaceutical consumption upon daily life.

The pharmaceuticalisation of daily life

According to business analysis, the pharmaceutical industry is the most profitable sector of commerce. Companies achieve profits of around 19 per cent of revenues while the top

10 corporations have a yield of 30 per cent of revenue (Angell 2000: 1902). In 2000, the global market for prescription drugs was $320 billion, and this figure is rising by about 10 per cent per year (Henry and Lexchin 2002). In this highly competitive field of endeavour, sustaining market share depends upon a mix of retaining existing business and development of new products, and while companies spend approximately 20 per cent of income on research and development, around 40 per cent is spent upon marketing (Angell 2000). Lifestyle drugs have contributed significantly to drug company profits during the past decade. In 1998, within three months of the approval of sildenafil in the US, Pfizer's profits jumped by 38 per cent (New York Times, 10 July 1998). Pfizer's 2006 annual report indicated sales stable at $1.7 billion per year, the company's fifth largest earner (Pfizer 2007). Orlistat, a significant earner for Roche with sales of just under $0.5 billion in 2005, was also licensed for over-the-counter (OTC) sales in 2006. Sanofi's new weight loss drug rimonabant (Acomplia) was heralded as a break-through chemical that might net $3 billion per year (Sargent 2006).

Applbaum (2006) has suggested that consumers are now a key element in the pharmaceutical 'distribution chain', alongside physicians, academic opinion leaders, patient advocacy groups, public health bodies and ethicists. This engagement transforms them from recipients of medical care to 'active consumers of the latest pharmaceuticals' (2006: 446, Fox and Ward 2006). In her analysis of female sexual dysfunction, Fishman (2004) notes the establishment of a direct connection between technology producers and consumers, mediated by DTC advertising, the commercialisation of self-help and consumer movements and the emergence of the Internet. These encourage an active consumerist perspective on health and health care, based on:

> the assumption that it is both the responsibility and the entitlement of the consumer/patient to find paths to better health (and in this case, better sex) through information gathering and through responsible consumption practices (Fishman 2004: 202)

In her essay on Viagra's impact on human sexuality, Marshall (2002: 133) argues that while drugs such as sildenafil have been adopted because they establish a molecular basis for an aspect of life such as sexuality, and are consequently accepted by professionals in medical and therapeutic communities as contributing to the 'natural sexual response cycle', a further critical element has been that they are accepted by consumers as a 'magic bullet' that will revolutionise sexual relations by restoring normal functionality. This suggests that the success of a drug rests not only in its capacity to achieve an effect, but on its interaction with cultural and social forces that define a condition as warranting a pharmaceutical resolution.[4] In our research, we found examples of how respondents confirmed the status of a drug, through their use of it but perhaps more importantly by their attribution of 'successful' resolution of a condition to its role. Richard had incorporated use of Viagra in his life, and accorded it significance for key aspects of his sexual relationship with his wife:

> I have ED all the time, as defined as the inability to achieve or maintain an erection. Does that mean do I always take a Viagra before I engage in sexual activity? No, I don't, because I engage my wife in some sort of sexual activity almost every day. She demands and deserves my physical attention. But when we want sustained intercourse, I take Viagra. That's maybe once or twice a week on average.

Another of our respondents, George, confirmed that using Viagra had become an integral element of his sexual life. Even though he had come to depend upon it, he accorded it accolades for resolving his ED problem:

> My best friend at the office introduced me to Viagra a week after he saw my attitude change at the office due to my noticeable depression. Thanks to Viagra, I felt I am gaining my manhood again, but now lazy of doing sex without the blue pill. I am now becoming a big fan of Viagra, and afraid of having sex without Viagra (George).

Similarly, users of Xenical had made the drug central to their diets, even though the main effect of the drug is simply to prevent fat uptake, not to control calories. Managing diet while taking the drug was tricky, in order to avoid the unpleasant side-effect of diarrhoea if fat was ingested, but Elsie regarded the drug, and not her own efforts to manage her diet, as the basis for her weight loss:

> If you eat a regular diet, separate your carbs from your fats and proteins, eat one carb meal and choose only coloured vegetables with your meats. The body metabolises better when you don't mix! I have also noticed that warm soups make Xenical work better. And fruit, it a great additive too (Elsie).

A weight loss drug, that she refers to as 'phen', had given Beth the sense that she need not simply depend on her own will-power. For her, the drug did assume the role of magic bullet (Marshall 2002: 133), the assistance she needed to keep to a diet:

> I know I needed help from phen, I could diet all I wanted, and still not lose, I could eat whatever I wanted, junk, fast food, and still not gain. I was stuck, I overate, I was depressed, and the day I ordered phen, I cancelled my doctor's appointment for getting depression meds. I wanted to give myself one more chance, and I have. Am I depressed, hell no, if anything I am now conceited, I love the mirror now and I don't care who knows it.

We can see elements of the pharmaceuticalisation of sexuality and weight loss within these extracts, as the drugs create a sensibility in which they become a core element of what goes on in their users' kitchens and bedrooms rather than something extraneous. Indeed, these respondents regard these pharmaceutical products as allies that have enabled them to overcome the physical restrictions of erectile dysfunction or obesity. The capacity of drugs such as sildenafil to generate such ardent fan bases confirm their success and assure the pharmaceuticalisation of the aspects of life they address.

Pharmaceutical companies have recognised the importance of consumer legitimation of their products, as reflected in their marketing strategies and target audiences. Newman (2006) described how the manufacturers of treatments for erectile dysfunction initially focused upon the treatment of disease, while negotiating approval with national governance bodies. Once established in these markets, both Pfizer (the manufacturer of sildenafil) and GlaxoSmithKline and Bayer (the makers of the rival vardenafil or Levitra) adopted popular sporting figures to front their marketing campaigns, re-focusing on a younger market by a mix of innuendo and machismo. Levitra was explicitly aimed at men who were sexually potent, but wanted 'to improve the quality or duration of their erections' (2006: 12). Lilly ICOS subsequently recruited actor Paul Newman as the face of Cialis, with a campaign aimed at both men and women (Newman 2006).

In our UK study, with direct advertising to consumers not an option, we found that pharmaceutical companies were working increasingly closely with patient groups such as breast cancer charities who wanted specific pharmaceuticals funded by insurance companies or state health services (Fox *et al.* 2005d). In their discussion of NHS funding of herceptin for breast cancer, Barrett *et al.* (2006: 1118) suggest that 'high profile patients, media bias, (and) industry support' were factors in persuading the National Institute for Health and Clinical Excellence (NICE) to approve the use of the drug in early stages of the disease. States and insurance schemes have often refused initially to subsidise consumers' payments for drugs that affect 'lifestyle', principally in order to control costs (Chisholm 1999). Unsurprisingly, by contrast, pharmaceutical companies are enthusiastic to get their drugs funded by these bodies to increase sales (for example, by NHS subsidy of prescriptions). However, decisions by a government to fund a product for certain categories of patient may depend upon defining a condition as pathological. This is true for sildenafil, which in the UK is now available on NHS prescription for men with erectile dysfunction (ED) arising from a range of underlying medical conditions and for those with the 'non-medical' diagnosis of 'severe distress' due to ED affecting mood, relationships or normal functioning (Sairam *et al.* 2002). Orlistat may be prescribed for those defined as overweight and for obese patients by body-mass index, but eligible patients must first have begun dietary, exercise and behavioural programmes to reduce weight (NICE 2006). Such funding decisions enhance the legitimacy both of the condition and the pharmaceutical agent that has been funded to treat it.

In this section we have demonstrated both micro- and macro-levels of activity around pharmaceutical products that contribute to a pharmaceuticalisation of daily life. We explore the interactions between these levels in the final section.

Discussion

We have argued that the pharmaceuticalisation of daily life entails both the application of pharmaceuticals to normalise specific lifestyle-related activities such as sex and body shape and the domestication of usage, and have offered examples from our own research and from the literature to illustrate these processes. We have also pointed out that the development and innovation of pharmaceuticals depends fundamentally upon the capacity of commercial businesses to turn a profit, and on their willingness to invest speculatively and massively in new products: to bring a new drug to market costs between $500 and $800 million for research, development and marketing, and takes approximately 12 years (Henry and Lexchin 2002: 1592). The industry has been criticised for focusing too heavily upon profitable and sometimes derivative new products (for example cholesterol-lowering drugs) rather than on drugs that will treat major illnesses, particularly those in newly developed countries where revenues will be limited (Angell 2000). This affects the commercial emphases within companies' research efforts, which necessarily focus on potential products that will sustain the levels of profits achieved historically. Where drugs are available, consumers may be unable to afford them, leading to some high-profile philanthropic deeds by drug companies anxious to avoid negative publicity (Henry and Lexchin 2002: 1590). As more products become available to treat aspects of daily life, access to a desired lifestyle outcome may depend increasingly upon individual or national resources.

While a profit motive underpins pharmaceutical production and consumption, there is a further link between individual choice and corporate decisions. As Fishman (2004) points out, pharmaceutical companies produce not only drugs but also the medico-scientific knowledge that justifies the product's value as the solution to a problem. Drugs such as sildenafil were promoted 'through scientific claims about the medical benefit, efficacy and necessity, supposedly revealed by objective clinical research' (2004: 189), with clinical trials serving not only to provide evidence of efficacy and safety, but also to legitimate products through an apparent separation between science and commercial interests. In the US, a drug can only gain Food and Drugs Administration (FDA) approval if it treats an established 'disease' (2004: 192), and consequently there will be strong efforts by manufacturers to biomedicalise lifestyle conditions. In Newman's (2006) analysis of US direct-to-consumer marketing of sildenafil, she notes that Pfizer were instrumental in getting the term erectile dysfunction or ED into common parlance, giving a medical-sounding spin to the condition previously know as impotence.

Other authors have reached similar conclusions about other drugs. Lexchin (2001: 1449) discusses the use of paroxetine (Seroxat or Paxil), which was licensed for the treatment of 'social phobia', a condition that elides into 'shyness', not previously regarded as a health problem. The availability of methylphenidate (Ritalin) may have hastened the acceptance of attention-deficit hyperactivity disorder (ADHD) as a medicalised description of disruptive behaviour in children (Fishman 2004: 193). Sleeplessness has similarly been accepted as a health problem, with remedies topping the US charts of consumer marketing spends of prescription drugs. The psychological consequences of androgenic alopecia (a secondary sexual characteristic that has been stigmatised since the time of the Roman Empire [Segrave 1996: 4]) may in time come to be regarded as pathological, perhaps as a form of 'body dysmorphic disorder', now that an effective drug treatment is available (Cash 2001: 163).

Not all efforts by pharmaceutical companies to pharmaceuticalise daily life have been successful, however. The winning formula of sildenafil and other ED drugs led Pfizer and other drug companies to search for 'pink Viagra' (Mayor 2004), a cognate drug that would address 'female sexual dysfunction' (FSD), a condition characterised by vaginal dryness, insufficient clitoral blood flow, lack of libido, sexual pain and inability to climax (Fishman 2004: 188, 194), and apparently affecting one woman in two (Laumann, Paik and Rosen 1999). The condition became the focus of interventions by a range of health and care professionals, of media attention, and of pharmaceutical innovation (Moynihan 2003). Yet despite considerable research efforts, the condition has remained recalcitrant to chemotherapy, although sildenafil is prescribed 'off-licence' for women on a case-by-case basis, as FSD is considered congruent with male sexual dysfunction (Fishman 2004: 199). Fishman (2002) notes that attention has now focused on women's brains (as opposed to their minds) as the target for a successful treatment for FSD, following the conclusion that arousal in women requires more than increased genital blood flow. If Marshall's (2002) evaluation of the requirements for a successful pharmaceutical treatment for an aspect of daily life is correct, then all that is now required is a suitable candidate chemical, as the willingness or desire by public and professionals to seek a pharmaceutical answer to the 'problem' of FSD seems assured, be it a 'real' or a constructed 'disease'.

From these examples we may conclude that the pharmaceuticalisation of daily life is a complex mix of factors that involves the biological effect of a chemical on human tissue, the legitimacy of a condition as a disease, the willngness of consumers to adopt the technology as a 'solution' to a problem in their lives, and the corporate interests of drug companies. Together, these factors contribute to the moulding of aspects of daily life into disease categories alongside the pharmaceutical agents that 'treat' them. Within the context of highly-invested daily life choices (for example, the ability to sleep through the night, or to have penetrative sex), drugs are ascribed potency and – as we saw in our data – replace the subject's own sense of themselves as agentic, becoming central to the lives of their users. It might appear that all parties are winners in this enterprise. However, the apparent benefits of these new treatments for problems of living may have been assumed. In a study of the female partners of Viagra users, Potts *et al.* (2003) point to the negative consequences of a ready treatment for erectile dysfunction. They found that the drug skewed couples' sexual activity towards penetration, often repeatedly over a prolonged period, as males wanted to get 'value for money'. This new emphasis was sometimes unwelcome, and could even lead to discomfort and injury. It had returned men to their pre-ED focus on penetrative sex at the expense of foreplay and other sexual activities (2003: 704). The drug had transformed their sex lives, but not for the better, as Viagra is:

> a socially-embedded phenomenon that not only affects a man's penis so that he may experience enhanced erectile capacity, but also affects his self-image, his lifestyle and his relationships with others in more personal ways. Moreover, Viagra is a device (or technology) which itself is coded with various social and cultural understandings about sexuality and masculinity (2003: 698–9).

The domestication of pharmaceutical consumption and the pharmaceuticalisation of life consequently affect the consumption of drugs associated with daily life, but perhaps more importantly the ways in which elements of our private lives are understood. In our research, we found that Viagra was taken for a wide range of motivations (Fox and Ward 2006), and similarly that weight loss pharmaceuticals were used to sustain anorexia (Fox *et al.* 2005b). We noted earlier Flower's (2004) definition of lifestyle use of pharmaceuticals as satisfying a 'non-health-related goal', but in the light of our analysis, we must ask exactly what counts as a 'non-health' use, when pharmaceutical companies lobby for new disease categories? We have seen that erectile dysfunction has come to be acknowledged as a medical problem, and in some circumstances pharmaceutical treatment is eligible for funding by states or under insurance schemes, even though the outcome is the 'lifestyle' objective of penetrative sex (Sairam *et al.* 2002). The domestication of pharmaceutical use, the 'lifestyle marketing' of a wider range of pharmaceutical products to physicians and users, the engagement of consumers and patient support groups within the distribution chain, and the co-option of scientific expertise to justify pharmaceuticals' raison d'etre, together contribute to a medicalisation of problems, experiences and perceptions that has no theoretical limits. Historians and anthropologists of medicine have shown how diseases appear and disappear in relation to contemporary theories and social processes (for example Figlio 1982, Maines 2001). In this chapter we have shown how the social relations surrounding contemporary pharmaceutical production and consumption link the world of business to the private worlds of citizens, forging new diseases and treatments from the very fabric of daily life.

Notes

1 ESRC grant L218252057, part of the Innovative Health Technologies programme.
2 When using online data, particularly to explore issues concerning embodiment, there is a need for some caution over interpretation. Online ethnography can limit the opportunities to evaluate the validity of data, in comparison with face-to-face interviews. Inevitably, the non-verbal clues that a researcher can use in interpretive methodologies will be missed where interactions are conducted in written media. Anonymity may increase intentional or unintentional deception (Glaser *et al.*

2002: 191) or identity manipulation (Hewson *et al.* 2003: 115). Participants need access to hardware, skills in typing and motivation to participate in what can be lengthy online interviews (Chen and Hinton 1999), and so may under-represent poor and minority groups, although Hewson *et al.* (2003: 32) consider that this bias is disappearing with increasing Internet access. Thomsen *et al.* (1998) suggest that multi-method triangulation using textual analysis, prolonged participant observation and qualitative interviews can provide valid and reliable data, and this is the approach we adopted. It remains a limitation of the design, however, that our participants may under-represent sectors of the community we are studying.

3 We thank an anonymous reviewer for this insight.
4 Both Castro-Vazquez (2006) and Hollander (2006) argue that approvals of drug treatments for erectile dysfunction reflect aspects of contemporary society, including social attitudes and norms concerning women's independence and sexual freedom, leading to fast-tracking approvals in comparison with contraceptives or abortion pharmaceuticals (see also Grimes 2004 on the approval of emergency contraceptives in the US).

References

Angell, M. (2000) The pharmaceutical industry – to whom is it accountable? *New England Journal of Medicine*, 342, 1902–4.

Applbaum, K. (2006) Pharmaceutical marketing and the invention of the medical consumer, *PLoS Medicine*, 3, 4, 445–7.

Barrett, A., Roques, T., Small, M. and Smith, R.D. (2006) How much will Herceptin really cost? *British Medical Journal*, 333, 1118–20.

Cash, T.F. (2001) The psychology of hair loss and its implications for patient care, *Clinics in Dermatology*, 19, 161–6.

Castro-Vazquez, R. (2006) The politics of Viagra: gender, dysfunction and reproduction in Japan, *Body and Society*, 12, 2, 109–29.

Chen, P. and Hinton, S.M. (1999) Realtime interviewing using the World Wide Web, *Sociological Research Online*, 4, 3 (Accessed at http://www.socresonline.org.uk/socresonline/4/3/chen.html).

Chisholm, J. (1999) Viagra: a botched test case for rationing, *British Medical Journal*, 318, 273–4.

Cockburn, C. (1994) The circuit of technology: gender, identity and power. In Silverstone, R. and Hirsch, E. (eds) *Consuming Technologies: Media and Information in Domestic Spaces*. London: Routledge.

Figlio, K. (1978) Chlorosis and chronic disease in 19th century Britain, *International Journal of Health Services*, 8, 589–617.

Fishman, J.R. (2002) Sex, drugs and clinical research, *Molecular Interventions*, 2, 1, 12–16.

Fishman, J.R. (2004) Manufacturing desire: the commodification of female sexual dysfunction, *Social Studies of Science*, 34, 2, 187–218.

Flower, R. (2004) Lifestyle drugs: pharmacology and the social agenda, *Trends in Pharmacological Sciences*, 25, 4, 182–5.

Fox, N.J. and Ward, K.J. (2006) Health identities: from expert patient to resisting consumer, *Health*, 10, 4, 461–79.

Fox, N.J., Ward, K.J. and O'Rourke, A.J. (2005a) 'Expert patients', pharmaceuticals and the medical model of disease: the case of weight loss drugs and the Internet, *Social Science and Medicine*, 60, 6, 1299–309.

Fox, N.J., Ward, K.J. and O'Rourke, A.J. (2005b) Pro-anorexia, pharmaceuticals and the Internet: resisting the medicalisation of body shape, *Sociology of Health and Illness*, 27, 7, 944–71.

Fox, N.J., Ward, K.J. and O'Rourke, A.J. (2005c) The birth of the E-Clinic. Continuity or transformation in the governance of pharmaceutical consumption? *Social Science and Medicine*, 61, 7, 1474–84.

Fox, N.J., Ward, K.J. and O'Rourke, A.J. (2005d) A sociology of technology governance for the information age: the case of pharmaceutical consumption, *Sociology*, 40, 2, 315–34.

General Accountability Office (2006) *Prescription Drugs*. Washington: US Government GAO (Accessed on 4 July 2007 at http://www.gao.gov/new.items/d0754.pdf).

Glaser, J., Dixit, J. and Green D. P. (2002) Studying hate crime with the Internet: what makes racists advocate racial violence? *Journal of Social Issues*, 58, 1, 177–92.

Grimes, D.A. (2004) Emergency contraception: politics trumps science at the U.S. Food and Drug Administration, *Obstetrics and Gynecology*, 104, 2, 220–1.

Haddon, L. (1994) Explaining ICT consumption: the case of the home computer. In Silverstone, R. and Hirsch, E. (eds) *Consuming Technologies: Media and Information in Domestic Spaces*. London: Routledge.

Henry, D. and Lexchin, J. (2002) The pharmaceutical industry as a medicines provider, *Lancet*, 360, 1590–95.

Hewson, C., Yule, P., Laurent, D. and Vogel, C. (2003) *Internet Research Methods*. London: Sage.

Hollander, I. (2006) Viagra's rise above women's health issues: an analysis of the social and political influences on drug approvals in the United States and Japan, *Social Science and Medicine*, 62, 683–93.

Laumann, E.O., Paik, A. and Rosen, R. (1999) Sexual dysfunction in the United States: prevalence and predictors, *Journal of the American Medical Association*, 281, 6, 537–44.

Lexchin, J. (2001) Lifestyle drugs: issues for debate, *Canadian Medical Association Journal*, 164, 10, 1449–51.

Maines, R.P. (2001) *The Technology of Orgasm: Hysteria, the Vibrator and Women's Sexual Satisfaction*. Baltimore: Johns Hopkins University Press.

Marshall, B.L. (2002) 'Hard science': gendered constructions of sexual dysfunction in the Viagra age, *Sexualities*, 5, 2, 131–58.

Mayor, S. (2004) Pfizer will not apply for a license for sildenafil for women, *British Medical Journal*, 328, 542.

Med Ad News Staff (2006) DTC takes a back seat, *Med Ad News*, May 2006 (Accessed on 4 July 2007 at http://www.pharmalive.com/magazines/medad/view.cfm?articleID=3522).

Mintzes, B. (2002) Direct to consumer advertising is medicalising normal human experience, *British Medical Journal*, 324, 908–11.

Moynihan, R. (2003) The making of a disease: female sexual dysfunction, *British Medical Journal*, 326, 45–7.

Moynihan, R., Heath, I. and Henry, D. (2002) Selling sickness: the pharmaceutical industry and disease-mongering, *British Medical Journal*, 324, 886–91.

Newman, R. (2006) 'Let's just say it works for me'. Rafael Palmeiro, major League Baseball, and the marketing of Viagra, *NINE: a Journal of Baseball History and Culture*, 14, 2, 1–14.

NICE (2006) *NICE Clinical Guideline 43: Obesity*. London: National Institute for Health and Clinical Excellence.

Ormrod, S. (1994) 'Let's make the dinner'. Discursive practices of gender in the creation of a new cooking process. In Silverstone, R. and Hirsch, E. (eds) *Consuming Technologies: Media and Information in Domestic Spaces*. London: Routledge.

Perdue, L. (2002) *Eroticabiz: how Sex Shaped the Internet*. Lincoln NE: iUniverse.

Pfizer Ltd (2007) *Annual Report 2006*. New York: Pfizer Worldwide Communications (Accessed at http://media.pfizer.com/pfizer/annualreport/2006/annual/review2006.pdf).

Potts, A., Gavey, N., Grace, V.N. and Vares, T. (2003) The downside of Viagra: women's experiences and concerns, *Sociology of Health and Illness*, 25, 7, 697–719.

Rheingold, H. (1995) *The Virtual Community*. London: Minerva.

Sairam, K., Kulinskaya, E., Hanbury, D. *et al.* (2002) Oral sildenafil (Viagra) in male erectile dysfunction: use, efficacy and safety profile in an unselected cohort presenting to a British district general hospital, *BMC Urology*, 2, 4.

Sargent, C. (2006) Sanofi diet pill may fatten sales on slim weight loss, *Bloomberg.com*, (29 June 2006) (Accessed on 4 July 2007 at http://www.bloomberg.com/apps/news?pid=20601085&sid=ahJCiwZZBWQQ&refer=europe).

Segrave, K. (1996) *Baldness. A Social History.* Jefferson, NC: McFarland.

Shakespeare, J., Neve, E. and Hodder, K. (2000) Is norethisterone a lifestyle drug? Results of database analysis, *British Medical Journal*, 320, 291.

Thomsen, S.R, Straubaar, J.D. and Bolyard, D.M. (1998) Ethnomethodology and the study of online communities: exploring the cyber streets, *Information Research*, 4, 1 (Accessed at http://informationr.net/ir/4-1/paper50.html).

5

Sociology of pharmaceuticals development and regulation: a realist empirical research programme
John Abraham

Introduction

The purpose of this chapter is to explain a theoretically and empirically rigorous framework within which sociology can progressively pursue searching research questions about 'pharmaceuticals and society'. In approaching the complex field of pharmaceuticals development and regulation, my strategy is first to articulate why a realist conceptualisation of interests is theoretically more coherent than apparently popular alternatives. For example, this involves the presupposition that pharmaceutical companies have objective interests in profit-maximisation, and that patients have objective interests in drugs having the maximum benefit-risk ratio possible. I then show why the necessity of that presupposition is validated by demonstrating that the rationale for the historical development of drug regulation only makes sense by appreciating that the health interests of consumers/patients cannot be reduced to their actions in the unregulated market.

Having established the existence of objective interests, I examine their precise relationships to regulatory developments using a synthesis of archival evidence from historical sociology and established theoretical models from political sociology. I argue that this relationship is best characterised by 'neo-liberal corporate bias' at the macro- and meso-levels of sociological analysis of political organisation and representation. Such bias is suggestive of, but does not determine, the nature of the micro-social processes of testing and regulating pharmaceuticals themselves. Yet no sociological analysis of pharmaceutical development and regulation would be complete without an investigation of those processes. I contend that, to investigate such micro-level processes adequately, one needs a realist sociology of scientific knowledge, which appreciates that the assessment of the validity of techno-scientific knowledge-claims is essential for their sociological explanation. Building on that methodological insight, I then outline how commercial interests have been shown to bias the science of drug testing and regulatory review away from the interests of patients and public health, in favour of the pharmaceutical industry.

Furthermore, to establish that this bias has had real adverse effects on the health of patients, I draw on international comparisons of drug regulation to demonstrate that drug injuries are not necessarily an inevitable by-product of technological progress in pharmaceuticals because some countries have fewer drug safety problems than others. Similarly, I marshal evidence to show that the lowering of techno-scientific standards for drug safety testing across the EU, US and Japan is not an inevitable price to be paid for faster development of therapeutically valuable medicines, but more plausibly a consequence of the internationalisation of neo-liberal corporate bias in pharmaceutical regulation. Based on these various bodies of evidence, I conclude that there is compelling evidence that, overall, neo-liberal corporate bias at the macro- and meso-levels of political organisation and representation leads to biases favourable to industry's and contrary to patients' interests at the micro-social level of science-based testing and regulating of drugs. Finally, I consider how biases against the interests of public health within pharmaceutical development and regulation could be reduced.

A realist framework of interests

Since the 1980s, the concept of 'interests' has become unfashionable in social sciences, giving way to a discourse of 'stakeholders' or 'fluid' 'actor-networks' (Adam *et al.* 2000, Rappert 2007). The attack on sociological explanations using a conceptualisation of interests came from within sociology and political commentary. For some, the idea that there could be objective interests consciously or unconsciously influencing the actions of people and organisations was challenged as an authoritarian meta-narrative (Bogard 1990, Dews 1987). Woolgar (1981: 37) asserted scathingly that such explanations of social action treated people as 'interest dopes'. He contended that 'there is no sense in which the phenomenon has an existence independent of its expression . . . there is no object beyond discourse . . . the organisation of discourse is the object' (Woolgar 1988: 73, 89). In other words, whatever actions or preferences people express *are* their interests, so the concept of 'interests' is superfluous (Potter 1996). Similarly, Schwarz and Thompson (1990) suggested that people's perspectives and commitments about say, drug safety, should be regarded as expressions of group political culture (or sub-culture), rather than identifiable interests (Hancher and Moran 1989).

These perspectives of what I call 'superficiality' coincided with an emerging sympathy for Hayekian writings about the appropriateness of the market for distributing resources and opportunities in society (Hayek 1967). The intelligibility of elevating the marketisation of society to such importance depended on the presupposition that people do not have interests beyond the preferences that they express in the market. The application of 'stake-holder' discourse reflected the application of this philosophy to the political process. Like consumers in a market, it was assumed that analysis could stop at stakeholders' expressed political preferences.[1] Indeed, rejecting 'interests' as fixed analytical categories capable of explanation, some commentators sought to define interests as nothing more than social actions and processes (Irwin 2001: 171).

I suggest that this is an impoverished view of sociological explanation. At a basic level of sociological theory, it is preferable to distinguish between actions/behaviour on the one hand, and interests on the other, because then it is possible to consider the possibility that people might behave against their own interests. That possibility cannot be discounted, in particular or in general, because a group's potential to act in its own interests is dependent on knowledge about how best to achieve particular goals – knowledge to which the group may have little or no access. In highly complex and functionally differentiated societies, such knowledge-deficits and dependencies are likely to be common, and always possible (Abraham and Davis 2007a).

Thus, it makes more sense for sociologists to employ a plausible framework of objective interests against which to examine the behaviour of various agents. Such a framework is based on the realist presupposition that there can be interests 'beyond' discourse and actions.[2] When considering the relationship between pharmaceuticals and society, I suggest that, to a first approximation, it is plausible to presuppose that an objective interest of patients and public health is that drugs released on to the market have the maximum possible benefit-risk ratio given all the scientific knowledge available at that time. Similarly, capitalist pharmaceutical companies have an objective, though not always over-riding, commercial interest in the maximisation of their profits.[3] This realist position is not merely an a priori fiat of sociological theory. It is borne out by historical sociology of the emergence of pharmaceutical regulation, which validates the plausibility of this realist theoretical framework of interests, as I show in the remainder of this section.

For many years pharmaceuticals escaped sociological scrutiny, not least because of the extremely limited conception of their links with 'society'. In late 19th and early 20th century Western industrialised countries, 'society' was little more than a market receptacle for the products of an expanding industry and profession of science and medicine. Few questioned the wisdom of doctors and scientists involved in the pharmaceutical trade. This permitted dominant producer interests to mobilise the powerful ideology[4] that the market could determine the best remedies for patients and health care (Abraham and Lewis 2002). On this view, the concept of 'interests' seemed insignificant because there was supposed to be a coincidence of interests between scientists, the medical profession and society – an ideology of coincidence of interests that was frequently promoted by drug manufacturers misinforming consumers about their products. All that mattered was that the drug trade, in collaboration with the scientific and medical professions, continued to progress with the production of more pharmaceuticals that consumers wanted to buy – because if consumers wanted to buy them then that must be in their interests. The first signs of the need to distinguish between the interests of the drug trade and consumers was when some manufacturers were accused of selling adulterated products. That is, consumers were being sold products of defective *quality* – they did not contain the ingredients they were supposed to (Abraham 1995a: 36–56).

By the early 20th century some government scientists and influential medical experts were campaigning for drug quality regulation to protect consumers' health against the dangers of drug adulteration. They were joined by the large, technologically sophisticated pharmaceutical firms, who saw an opportunity to close out competition from other drug traders because the large companies could easily meet the expected new regulatory standards, while other drug producers could not. This coalition was successful in bringing about the introduction of drug-quality regulation. Evidently, the interests of consumers and the drug trade did not always coincide. As doctors retreated from the manufacture of drugs, the drug trade fragmented between companies concentrating on the production of drugs for prescription by doctors (known as 'ethical pharmaceuticals') and the firms who marketed their products directly to consumers (Barkan 1985, Stieb 1966).

While drug quality was subject to government regulation there continued an assumption that the techno-science of the 'ethical' pharmaceutical industry could be trusted to provide safe and effective medicines. Patients' interests were subsumed by the industry's as it was argued by industry and governments that it was not in firms' commercial interests to produce unsafe or ineffective drugs. However, pharmaceutical companies' commercial interests in the market proved a very poor barometer for drug safety or efficacy as demonstrated by drug disasters and thousands of products found to be ineffective when eventually tested independently of the industry (Abraham 1995a: 56–74). While pharmaceutical firms did not want drug disasters, their commercial interests evidently did not coincide sufficiently with those of patients to investigate thoroughly enough drugs of dubious safety.

Consequently, between the late 1920s and the mid-1970s, all the Western industrialised countries introduced government regulation of drug safety and efficacy, as well as quality. For the first time, only *government* agencies had the legal authority to determine whether a new drug was safe and effective enough to be permitted on to the market. The timing of such regulation varied from 1928 in Norway, 1935 in Sweden, 1962 in the US, and 1971 in the UK, to 1976 in (West) Germany (Abraham 1995a: 36–86, Abraham and Lewis 2000: 49–76).

Hence, governments came to regulate drug quality, safety and efficacy purportedly on behalf of patients and public health. Governments accept that it is their legal responsibility to protect the interests of patients in these respects. Evidently, therefore, the rationale for the historical emergence of pharmaceutical regulation demonstrates that the health interests of patients and the wider public reside *beyond* the preferences and desires that consumers or patients express in either the market or the political process. Moreover, the explanation for the disjuncture between patients' interests and their expressed desires in the market and clinic often resided in the ideological creation of false consciousness about pharmaceuticals, due to misleading drug promotion by companies and lack of comprehensive public access to accurate information about drug risks and benefits (Abraham and Sheppard 1997, Chetley 1990: 51–68, Collier 1989: 75–87, Medawar 1979). Thus, there are not only a priori reasons to support a realist framework of interests; there are also empirical historical ones. Indeed, as the foregoing account demonstrates, one cannot make sense of the history of drug regulation without such a framework.

Political sociology of regulation: corporate bias, neo-liberalism and capture

The previous section shows that, despite current fashions, the appreciation of the existence of objective interests is indispensable for our sociological understanding of pharmaceutical regulation. That realisation, however, conveys nothing about the *specific* relationships between interests and regulatory developments. To address this empirical matter, I turn to political sociology, which is often mistaken for a purely theoretical sub-discipline. However, there is an empirical branch of political sociology concerned with testing theories of political actors and organisations. Here, we are particularly concerned with how theories of the regulatory state, such as capture theory, corporatism and neo-liberalism, relate to empirical findings about macro- and meso-level politics of regulatory development throughout history. Probably the best known theory of regulation is that of regulatory capture epitomised by the 'life-cycle' theory of regulatory agencies put forward by Bernstein (1955). On this view, regulatory agencies are set up by the legislature in order to protect the public interest against the excesses of industrial power. It is assumed that there exists some divergence, if not conflict, of interests between industry, seeking to maximise profits, and 'the public interest'.

Initially, regulatory agencies tend to be adversarial towards industry, but become isolated as their enthusiastic staff tire and retire. Eventually, they are progressively 'captured' by, and come to share the perspectives of, the industries they are supposed to regulate. Regulatory capture may result from direct industry lobbying of government officials, co-opting expert advisors to regulatory agencies by giving them grants or consultancies, or the 'revolving door' signalling that regulatory officials begin their careers in industry, then work for some years in the regulatory agency until they are promoted back into the higher echelons of industry (Braithwaite 1984: 298, Hancher and Moran 1989b: 288, Owen and Braeutigam 1978). According to capture theory, if regulators have trained in industry and/or they see their career development in terms of future promotion into the regulated industry, then they may be unduly concerned to maintain 'friendly relations' with industry at the expense of public interest regulation From this captured stage onwards, argues Bernstein, the regulatory agency prioritises industrial interests over consumers, unless, or until, a scandal highlighting the failures of regulation triggers a new drive for public interest regulation, in which case the regulatory agency begins a new cycle.

Theories of regulatory capture assume that, at the outset, regulation was established in order to serve the public interest (Mitnick 1980). By contrast, corporatist theory envisages a more pro-active regulatory state with its own interests. Unlike capture theory, regulatory agencies do not evolve cyclically between solely protecting the 'public interest' (before capture) and passively defending industry interests (after capture). Corporatist theories propose that the nature of regulatory systems is shaped by organised interests, together with two-way bargaining between those interests and the interests of the state (Cawson 1986). Some interests are more organised than others, and are capable of gaining exceptional influence over the regulatory state because of their (near) monopoly over resources needed for regulation. For example, in the pharmaceutical sector, regulation might be characterised as corporatist because the industry's possession of 'reservoirs of expertise' implies that its integration into the implementation of the regulatory process is virtually a pre-condition for its success, rather than a result of capture (Hancher and Moran 1989: 272). On the other hand, a neo-liberal regulatory state would be expected to be minimal and subject to the tests of 'the market' (Boreus 1997).

Extensive archival research covering the last hundred years or so has been conducted on the political sociology of pharmaceutical regulation in the US, UK, the EU and other European countries (Abraham 2007). The evidence supports what I call 'corporate bias' (a variant of corporatism consistent with some indicators of capture) up to the 1980s and subsequently 'neo-liberal corporate bias', rather than pure corporatism, capture or neo-liberalism. By 'corporate bias' I mean that the pharmaceutical industry was, and is, permitted to have privileged strategic access to, and involvement with, government regulatory policy over and above any other interest group; and more often than other factors, the industry was, and is, decisive in determining regulatory policy outcomes (or lack thereof). The regulatory state and the pharmaceutical industry work largely in partnership and behind a cloak of secrecy.

Corporate bias is the preferred characterisation over regulatory capture because regulatory agencies and reforms were not instigated solely or largely in response to public campaigns for better drug quality, safety and testing in the public interest. Such campaigns either came to nothing in the way of regulatory reform or contributed only to belated and diluted regulatory change unless they also had support from the industry or the state itself. For example, in the UK, this is well documented with respect to: (1) the anti-adulteration campaigns of the 1880s and 1890s; (2) regulatory inaction in the aftermath of the 1914 Select Committee's recommendations for strict regulations governing the therapeutic claims made by pharmaceutical manufacturers of 'patent medicines';[5] (3) the fact that, despite clearly knowing about the 1937 Elixir Sulfanilimide drug disaster in the US, which killed 107 people and ushered in US drug safety regulation (1938), there is no trace of any reform efforts at all within the Ministry of Health to introduce government regulation of drug safety in Britain in response to this disaster, even though it could just as easily have occurred in the UK; (4) the 1941 Pharmacy and Medicines Act, which brought incidental consumer protection by putting an end to 'patent medicines', but was motivated by the changing commercial interests of the industry, rather than the protection of public health; and (5) the 10-year delay between thalidomide (1961) and the implementation of legally enforceable drug safety regulation in 1971 under the *1968 Medicines Act* (Abraham 1995a: 36–86).

While many of the socio-political indicators of a 'captured' regulatory agency are endemic within pharmaceutical regulation, they do not evolve in a progressive cycle towards industrial capture of public interest regulation. Rather, the pharmaceutical industry's privileged influence is evident at the outset of regulatory developments. For this reason also, corporate bias is a better account of pharmaceutical regulation than capture theory. In the UK, some examples of the pharmaceutical industry's privileged access to government in the *formation* of regulation are: (1) its moulding of the perspective of the Ministry of Health since the latter's inception in 1919; (2) its shaping of the voluntary Committee on Safety of Drugs (1963–68) and the *1968 Medicines Act*, especially the policy

Table 1 *Percentage of industry fee contribution to total EMEA budget and to FDA spending on human drug review*

Year	Percentage of total EMEA revenues*	Percentage of FDA spending on drug review**
1994		24
1995	28	36
1996	38	36
1997	48	36
1998	53	40
1999	70	43
2000	71	47
2001	69	50
2002	64	47
2003	67	49

Sources: *Figures for EMEA compiled from EMEA Annual Reports between 1995 and 2003. **Figures for FDA compiled from 65 Federal Register 47994 and annual financial reports to Congress from 2000.

that commercial secrecy took priority over provision of information to the public and wider medical/scientific community; and (3) its effective power to veto the Department of Health's proposal in 1970 that members of the Government's expert Committee on Safety of Medicines (CSM), which advised on whether new pharmaceuticals were safe and efficacious enough to be permitted and kept on the market, should be prohibited from having personal and non-personal interests in pharmaceutical companies, such as shareholding and consultancies (Abraham 1995a: 36–86, Abraham and Lewis 2002).

Furthermore, capture theory cannot accommodate the fact that at various times the regulatory state has been concerned with its own viability to the extent of defining its own interests independent of the industry and wider public. In the UK, this is evident from: the introduction of the *1920 Dangerous Drugs Act* to discipline public order; the black-listing of NHS drugs, which lacked proof of therapeutic value, by the Joint Committee on Prescribing in the 1950s in order to rationalise the costs of pharmaceuticals to the Service; and the 'Limited List' introduced by the Government in 1984 which excluded about 1,800 pharmaceutical preparations that the NHS would no longer pay for because they were judged to be too expensive and of little therapeutic advantage to patients (Abraham 1995a, Abraham and Sheppard 1999a, Gabe and Bury 1988).

There is extensive evidence that the corporate bias of pharmaceuticals regulation has taken on a neo-liberal flavour since the 1980s. Since 1989 the funding of the UK drug regulatory agency has changed from being derived 40 per cent from direct taxation to being 100 per cent derived from fees from pharmaceutical companies. Subsequently, many other European countries have very substantially increased the financial dependence of their drug regulatory agencies on fees from pharmaceutical companies – fees whose payment accompanies the drugs that the companies submit to the regulatory agencies for approval (Abraham and Lewis 2000: 43–79). In the EU and the US, such funding has grown steadily from the mid-1990s to reach about 70 per cent for the European Medicines Evaluation Agency (EMEA) and 50 per cent for the Food and Drug Administration (FDA) (Table 1). Thus, the regulatory state has become increasingly minimalist, that is, its independent resource-base is shrinking.

This has created a situation in which the institutional prosperity and viability of regulatory agencies depends on their ability to attract fees from pharmaceutical firms. Consequently,

Table 2 *FDA review* and approval** times for priority and standard NMEs, 1993–2003*

Calendar year	Priority			Standard		
	Number approved	Median FDA review time (months)	Median total approval time (months)	Number approved	Median FDA review time (months)	Median total approval time (months)
1993	13	13.9	14.9	12	27.2	27.2
1994	12	13.9	14.0	9	22.2	23.7
1995	10	7.9	7.9	19	15.9	17.8
1996	18	7.7	9.6	35	14.6	15.1
1997	9	6.4	6.7	30	14.4	15.0
1998	16	6.2	6.2	14	12.3	13.4
1999	19	6.3	6.9	16	14.0	16.3
2000	9	6.0	6.0	18	15.4	19.9
2001	7	6.0	6.0	17	15.7	19.0
2002	7	13.8	16.3	10	12.5	15.9
2003	9	6.7	6.7	12	13.8	23.1

*Review times are defined as the total time involved while the application is with the FDA for review. **Approval time is review time plus any time waiting for the company to make revisions that are pre-conditions for approval. *Source*: FDA – available at http://www.fda.gov

regulatory agencies are encouraged to compete by making themselves attractive to drug companies, who have come to be defined as the regulators' 'customers'. In effect, the drug regulatory agencies compete with each other on a market selling their regulatory services to pharmaceutical companies. As the customers (the drug firms) want rapid drug approval, the speed of regulatory agencies' regulatory review times has become the central criterion of this competition (Abraham and Lewis 1999). In short, the drug regulatory agencies have been subjected to the 'tests of the market' – another hallmark of neo-liberalism. As shown in Table 2, regulatory review times for new patentable drugs, known as new molecular entities (NMEs) in the US have been cut by half since 1993 and these reductions are based on previous cuts since the early 1990s (Kaitin and DiMasi 2000, Kessler *et al.* 1996). Similar trends have occurred in Europe. For example, the average net in-house review times of the UK regulatory agency for new drugs fell from 154 working days in 1989 to just 44 days by 1998. The regulatory review times of Germany, Sweden and many other EU countries also fell dramatically in this period (Abraham and Lewis 2000: 20).

Such inter-agency competition is particularly acute in European countries and other small to medium-sized markets. It has always been less so in the US because, with such a large market, trans-national pharmaceutical companies are generally keen to apply to the FDA anyway. However, the international competitive pressure on the FDA to accelerate its regulatory review consequent upon increased industry funding is present by a different mechanism. The FDA was subject to severe budgetary cuts during the Reagan Administrations, which reduced the number of employees from 8,200 in 1979 to 7,000 in 1987. Over the same period Congress had passed 20 new laws giving the FDA new responsibilities in both the food and drug area (Anon 1989). The Bush (senior) Administration, in its turn, continued to hold down FDA budgets (Hilts 2003: 255). To avert budgetary disaster the pharmaceutical industry agreed to part fund the agency via users' fees under the *1992 Prescription Drug Users Fee Act (PDUFA)* and subsequent renewals of the Act every five years, but only in exchange for explicit acceleration of regulatory review defined by industry demands.

In this context, the FDA also finds itself competing with other drug regulatory agencies for fastest review times because it is compared with them when industry and Congress review its funding every five years. Indeed, speed of regulatory review is now the primary quantitative performance indicator for the agency. It is sometimes argued that these accelerations of regulatory review in Europe and the US have been driven by patients and have then implied that this is in the interests of public health (Carpenter 2004, Daemmrich and Krucken 2000). *Sometimes*, especially in the early stages of AIDS patient activism, there is *some* truth in this.[6] However, these regulatory reforms have for the most part made no attempt to prioritise the interests of patients' health.[7] For example, the demands on the FDA to speed up its regulatory reviews apply to standard drugs, which offer little or no therapeutic advance, as well as to priority drugs, while in Europe, regulatory agencies do not even collect the requisite data to routinely distinguish between standard and priority drugs in the first place (Abraham and Davis 2007b).

Science, drug development and product regulation in the post-thalidomide era

So far I have discussed the (neo-liberal) corporate bias of political *organisation* and *representation* in pharmaceutical regulation. While this is suggestive of commercial bias and other influences on the actual testing and regulation of drug products themselves, such micro-level processes must be empirically researched in order to establish the effects of (neo-liberal) corporate bias on regulatory science, decision making and outcomes. The pharmaceutical industry conducts all the testing of its own drugs, and government regulatory agencies review the technical data submitted by the companies before deciding whether drugs can be approved for marketing as safe and effective.

Drug testing and regulatory review is conducted by scientists, drawing on fields such as biochemistry, toxicology, pharmacology, clinical pharmacology and pharmaco-epidemiology. Typically, such scientists deny that their assessments and knowledge-claims are biased by commercial or other political interests. A challenge for sociology was, and remains, to determine how social factors, such as interests, may influence and bias scientific knowledge-claims in drug testing and regulation. In short, a sociology of scientific knowledge (SSK) was required and an understanding of this sub-discipline within sociology had to be mobilised.

The pioneers of SSK had developed a number of valuable techniques, such as the examination of scientific controversies as a way of eliciting the roles of values and interests in science (Collins 1981). However, they located their analyses within a relativist-constructivist framework, which assumed that truth-value itself was merely a social construction. On this view, knowledge-claims were not structured by a mind-independent natural world, but rather what science told us about nature was the product of the values, subcultures and interests of the scientists involved. As Collins and Yearley (1992: 310) note, the self-proclaimed effect of this relativist constructivism 'has been to show that the apparent independent power of the natural world is granted by human beings in social negotiation'.

Reflecting this perspective, relativist-constructivists promoted the methodological canon of 'symmetry' in SSK, that is, the assumption that 'true' and 'false' beliefs are held to have equivalent types of sociological explanation (Bloor 1973, Collins 1995). Scientific knowledge-claims became scientific knowledge*s* because, argued relativist-constructivists, there was no objective reality against which to test the validity of knowledge-claims. For relativist-constructivists, when there was scientific controversy, this was to be characterised as no more than a *difference* in 'world-view' or sub-cultural values. One knowledge-claim could be regarded as superior to another only by reference to the instrumental goals of the actors involved, but there was no objective basis upon which to judge between knowledge-claims *beyond* such shared goals (Knorr-Cetina and Mulkay 1983: 6). In short, for constructivists there were multiple realities and multiple knowledges, that is, knowledge became (inappropriately) collapsed into belief.

Hence, such relativism limited itself to descriptions of how scientists constructed their knowledge-claims, but permitted the validity of knowledge-claims to escape scrutiny on both epistemological and methodological grounds. Furthermore, when subjected to the relativist (and social science) principle of reflexivity, relativist-constructivists' descriptions of science become devoid of any defensible criteria of validity. As Collins and Yearley (1992: 302) put it, such relativism 'opened up new ways of knowing nothing'. Unfortunately, therefore, relativist constructivism, if faithfully applied, renders the project of knowledge-production in sociology and social science unintelligible. While this relativist-constructivist approach to SSK is clearly inadequate, it is entirely unnecessary.

By contrast, the realist empirical research programme in SSK presupposes that knowledge-claims in science are the combined product of the social organisation of scientists *and* a mind-independent natural reality. It follows from this that the truth-value of scientific knowledge-claims is not merely the result of scientists' social constructions; it is also, in part, determined by the objective structure of the natural world. Hence, the explanation for 'true' beliefs may be of a very different type from 'false' beliefs because the main explanation for the former may be that it accurately accounts for a natural mechanism (*e.g.* hydrogen combined with oxygen produces water), while that cannot be the case for 'false' beliefs. That is to say, there is asymmetry. In addition, the realist empirical research programme in SSK is robustly reflexive because it appreciates that, just as scientists can discover truths about the natural world (with more or less accuracy), sociologists can discover truths about the social world (with more or less accuracy).

Thus, the sociological investigation of scientific knowledge needs to take into account the validity of knowledge-claims, if only to appreciate the asymmetrical nature of explanation concerning the role of social factors in producing 'true' and 'false' claims. Once it is appreciated that the validity of scientific knowledge-claims is important for SSK, then it immediately follows that the sociology of bias in science is also important. In this context, bias is defined as a consistent trend or pattern of technical inconsistencies or contradictions mapped on to a set of social interests. As demonstrated by the realist empirical programme in SSK, technical inconsistencies can take many forms. For example, contradictions between: how scientists test a drug in practice and the standards supposed to be upheld in their science at that time; what the same scientist says about a drug product in different contexts; the technical standards that regulators are supposed to be upholding and actual regulatory decisions; and contradictions between the standards applied to different scientists investigating the same drug (Abraham 1993, 1994, 1995b, Van Zwanenberg and Millstone 2000).

At any particular time in pharmaceutical development and regulation there are techno-scientific regulatory standards, whose publicly declared purpose is to protect and promote public health by ensuring that drug products are adequately safe and efficacious. Methodologically, those standards can be deployed by sociologists to investigate how well, in practice, pharmaceutical testing and regulation act in the interests of public health, and how far they are influenced by commercial or other interests. Claims and practices that are inconsistent with such standards provide a starting point for sociological investigation of whether drug testing and regulation is being biased away from the interests of patients and public health and, therefore, in contradiction to its publicly declared social function.[8] The realist empirical research programme has demonstrated that there has indeed been such a bias in modern pharmaceutical regulatory science since the 1970s – a claim yet to be contradicted by the pharmaceutical industry, government regulators, expert scientists, academic social scientists or lawyers, who have all aggressively reviewed it. Those biases are deeply embedded in complex ideologies about drug safety and pharmaceutical innovation, to which I now turn.

International comparisons and the ideology of drug safety

International comparison has also proved a valuable method in the micro-level sociology of pharmaceuticals by sharpening analyses of whose interests are served by the different socio-political arrangements that influence the approaches and outcomes of regulatory science in different countries. Two types of international difference have been scrutinised: differences in pre-market approval/evaluation of drug safety and efficacy of individual drug products; and differences in trends of post-market withdrawals of drug products on safety grounds. To date, most of these comparisons have been between the US and the UK or other European countries.

This longitudinal sociological research has shown that between 1971 and 1992 there were twice as many drug safety withdrawals in the UK as in the US because the FDA undertook more rigorous pre-market regulatory review, identified the safety problems and so never approved the drugs in the first place (Abraham and Davis 2005a). Meanwhile, the drugs were approved in the UK and caused drug injury to patients there until they were removed from the market. This realist comparative research has corrected a number of fallacious ideologies about UK drug safety regulation that had carried some sway. For example, UK regulators, industry representatives and many media commentators had argued that the level of drug safety withdrawals in the UK was unavoidable because of the unpredictability of drug safety (Abraham and Davis 2006). They also claimed that the UK's regulatory policy of 'early licensing' (with minimal pre-market regulatory checks) was compatible with the interest of patients because the UK had such a good post-market drug safety surveillance system that drugs could be withdrawn rapidly if safety problems occurred (Abraham and Davis 2005b). These technical arguments, however, were shown to be invalid because the FDA detected many of the safety problems from pre-market data, and when there were safety problems with drugs approved in the US, the FDA typically withdrew them much faster than the UK (Abraham and Davis 2005a). That the determination of the (non-)validity of those arguments contributes to the correcting of insights into the interests of regulatory science is one example of why an examination of the validity of technical knowledge-claims must be included in sociological analysis, rather than evaded.

Sociological comparisons of case studies confirmed the extent to which the FDA had tended to demand greater assurances from pharmaceutical firms about both drug safety and efficacy than their UK counterparts in this period before marketing approval. Furthermore, they indicated that the explanations were multi-faceted. Compared with the highly secretive system of British drug regulation, there was much greater freedom of information about drug regulation in the US, so the FDA was propelled into a situation of greater public accountability; there was regular legislative oversight by the Congress to investigate the FDA's performance in regulating drugs to protect public health. Furthermore, the public health advocacy organisations specialising in pharmaceuticals are much larger and more active, and the courts are much more active in reviewing the adequacy of drug testing and regulation, especially with respect to drug injury to patients (Abraham 1995a). These socio-political arrangements militated in favour of regulation in the interests of public health and attenuated the biasing influences of commercial interests on regulatory science.

More recent case-study comparisons of EU drug regulation and the FDA suggest that between 1995 and 2005 the differences between the regulatory demands of the FDA and the UK/EU have shrunk. Significantly, in this later period, Congressional oversight of the FDA has switched to an emphasis on acceleration of drug approvals rather than protection of patients from unsafe or ineffective drugs. Moreover, the implementation of US freedom of information legislation has been allowed to deteriorate by starving it of resources so that citizens may have to wait up to a year for a substantial response. Thus, the convergence of regulatory standards on both sides of the Atlantic tends to confirm previous sociological explanations as the convergence is mainly due to the FDA's weakening demands on pharmaceutical firms, which is in turn a result of the reversal or absence of social factors that previously explained the FDA's more demanding regulatory review than its UK and European counterparts (Abraham and Davis 2007b).

Importantly, the case studies of pharmaceutical testing and regulation not only revealed international differences in the extent to which pharmaceutical companies and regulatory agencies behaved in accordance with the declared purpose of their science. They also demonstrated biases and the influence of commercial interests in drug testing and regulation *within* each of the countries researched. Even when the FDA acted to protect the interests of public health more than its UK counterparts, its regulatory decisions were not necessarily unaffected by biasing influences from commercial interests. For example, the FDA required many more regulatory checks on the safety and efficacy of the anti-arthritis drug, benoxaprofen, and approved it much later, than the UK regulatory authorities. The agency, however, still approved the drug, which was to be a disaster, despite many *evident* toxicities and problems with efficacy data *before* approval (Abraham 1995a).

Streamlining global standards and the ideology of pharmaceutical innovation

By the early 1990s, the cost of bringing a new molecular entity (NME) to the market could be as high as US$350 million and it is estimated that the time from first synthesis of a new drug to its marketing quadrupled between 1960 and 1989 (Halliday *et al.* 1997: 63, Tansey *et al.* 1994: 85). In response, the industry strove to decrease the cost and duration of R and D by reducing regulatory requirements imposed by the state, and to reach larger markets more effectively. Such transnational firms could get better returns on R and D investments if they could access international markets simultaneously (McIntyre 1999: 96). Hence, during the 1990s the pharmaceutical industry sought to persuade regulatory agencies to harmonise regulatory standards for drug testing across geographical regions and to streamline the standards demanded.

To this end the International Federation of Pharmaceutical Manufacturers' Associations (IFPMA) established the International Conference on Harmonisation of Technical Requirements for Registration of Pharmaceuticals for Human Use (ICH) in 1990. The key participants in ICH are the three pharmaceutical industry associations and the three government drug regulatory agencies of the EU, Japan and the US. With IFPMA acting as Secretariat, the ICH met regularly throughout the 1990s and 2000s to agree changes to regulatory standards across the three regions that they claimed would not undermine patient safety. However, sociological studies have shown that many of these changes reduced the standards of testing that pharmaceutical companies had previously been required to meet on chronic toxicity testing, carcinogenicity testing, patient exposure during clinical risk assessment and reporting of adverse drug reactions (Abraham and Reed 2001, 2002, 2003). In this respect, these changes were in the commercial interests of the industry, but consistently inconsistent with the interests of patients and public health because new drugs would enter the market with fewer safety checks than before. On the other hand, this biased regulatory science was justified on the grounds that such streamlining of drug testing would deliver more pharmaceutical innovation needed by patients. The secretariat of the ICH contended that 'the urgent need' for harmonisation was 'impelled' by 'the need to meet the public expectation that there should be a minimum of delay in making safe and efficacious treatments available to patients in need', and to accelerate the development of 'life-saving treatments' and 'ground-breaking treatments of the future' (IFPMA 1998, 2000: 1).

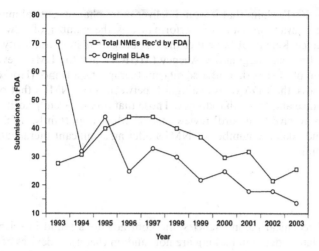

Figure 1 *10-year trends in major drug and biological product submissions to FDA.*
Source: FDA – available at http://www.fda.gov/oc/initiatives/criticalpath/nwoodcock0602.html

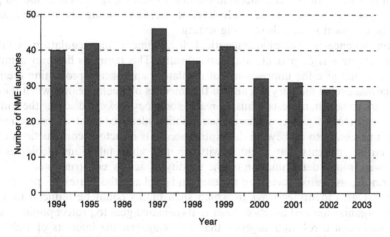

Figure 2 *Number of NMEs first launched onto the world market (1994–2003)*
NMEs = new molecular entities; BLAs = biologicals licence applications
Source: Centre for Medicines Research (2005)

A clear sociological problem is whether this promise of innovation is best regarded as a fallacious ideology or a reasonable account of the reality of the relationship between pharmaceutical innovation and patient need. Because the ICH's claims for innovation are futuristic and open-ended in time, one cannot provide a clear-cut answer to this problem. What can be said is that, despite the enormous neo-liberal acceleration of regulatory approval times in the last 20 years and the reductions in safety testing requirements via ICH in the last 15 years, pharmaceutical innovation has been declining over the last decade world wide, as measured by numbers of new molecular entities (NMEs) and original biologicals (*e.g.* vaccines) submitted to regulatory agencies and/or launched on to the world market (Figures 1 and 2).

Regarding the ICH's claim that it would deliver more pharmaceutical innovation *needed* by patients, the relevant measure of performance is the number of new drugs offering therapeutic advance. Remarkably, neither the UK drug regulatory authority, the Medicines and Healthcare Products Regulatory Agency (MHRA), nor the EMEA even collect data on the proportion of NMEs that offer significant therapeutic advance (House of Commons 2005). Nevertheless, the FDA does distinguish between those NMEs that offer significant therapeutic advance and those that do not. Those that do are given 'priority' review status, while the others receive 'standard' review status.[9] Most importantly, Table 2 shows that between 1993 and 2003 the number of NMEs offering significant therapeutic advance has also been declining.

Conclusion

The micro-level technical inconsistencies and contradictions found in science-based drug testing and regulatory decision making are not random rhetorical devices of isolated social contexts/practices as relativist-constructivists would have us believe. With sustained sociological endeavour, they can be systematically linked to objective interests, whose relationship with pharmaceutical regulation may be best characterised as neo-liberal corporate bias. Such bias in political organisation at the macro- and meso-levels does indeed produce biases in regulatory science at the micro-level of decision making about individual drugs and specific technical standards for drug testing.

The consequence is that pharmaceutical development and regulation is failing to maximise the interests of patients and public health. This failure is however camouflaged by ideologies that give the impression that regulatory approaches promoting the interests of the pharmaceutical industry are also in the interests of public health, when they are, in fact, contrary to health interests. Thus, as realist sociology seeks to discover the truth about how well regulatory agencies achieve their publicly declared goal of protecting public health, it is necessary to go beyond descriptive accounts of actors' constructions of reality – constructivist accounts that might unwittingly reproduce fallacious ideologies because they shy away from a determination of the validity of actors' constructions.

Furthermore, as realist sociology exposes and explains the biases of pharmaceutical regulation, it also identifies ways in which such biases could be reduced by bringing regulatory organisation and practice closer to its declared goal to protect public health. For example, sociological research suggests that biases against the interests of public health could be counteracted by a number of measures. Comprehensive public rights of access to regulatory information and timely public accountability of regulatory decision making could be introduced. There could be state funding of regulatory agencies that is entirely independent of the pharmaceutical industry and sufficient to enforce rigorous standards of accuracy regarding industry product promotion, combined with a separation of the science of drug testing from the industry for at least some pivotal tests. Such tests could be conducted by government regulatory scientists. In addition, a prohibition of expert regulatory scientists from having any personal financial interests in pharmaceutical companies would be desirable. Then, there is the need for regular and pro-active legislative oversight which could ensure that drug regulatory agencies are progressing towards their ostensible constitutional goal to protect public health. Finally, there could be readily available access for patients to judicial review of the conduct of pharmaceutical companies to ensure their accountability to the interests of public health beyond the reviewing processes of regulatory agencies.

Notes

1 The concept of 'stakeholders' replaced the concept of 'interest groups' in much of social science discourse in publications, grant applications and conference proceedings. That substitution implied a dis-association from a theoretical perspective committed to the view that interests underpinned social relations and beliefs. Use of 'stakeholder discourse' by many social scientists (wittingly or unwittingly) implied that, at the very least, there was not necessarily a need to locate actors within a framework of objective interests. Typically, the role of interests is not explicitly or reflexively defined in stakeholder discourse, but implicitly it seems that interests are to be empirically recorded as (no more than) stakeholders' expression of their goals and desires. Of course, hypothetically, one could retrospectively define stakeholders as 'actors with interests', but that renders the concept of 'stakeholders' redundant because then one might just as well revert to the concept of 'interest groups'.

2 It might be argued that the 'superficiality' perspective 'brings more rather than less "reality" to the issue' because it involves empirical studies of actions (Irwin 2001: 166–67). But realists also employ empirical studies seeking to explain, as well as recount, actions. Moreover, Irwin's argument is analogous to saying that if the highway code were an impoverished document, then that flaw could be set aside so long as the authors did plenty of driving!

3 Space constraints prevent a more differentiated discussion of interests. As one moves from the macro to meso and micro levels of analysis, different interests may be specified.

4 By 'ideology' I mean a set of beliefs that distort reality.

5 'Patent medicines' were 'secret remedies', whose ingredients were not disclosed on the label to patients/consumers.

6 In some cases, patient groups press for early release of new drugs as a 'last resort', though the extent to which this is a major driver of regulatory problems and reforms has been exaggerated, compared with other factors, by the media and some social scientists (Abraham and Sheppard 1999b). If a number of patients on a drug trial in such circumstances have benefited and they wish to continue on the drug, even though the trial's overall evidence-base shows no therapeutic benefit/efficacy, then it may be in the interests of that minority of patients to have continued access to the drug. A policy response consistent with the interests of those patients is to permit continued 'compassionate' release of the drug to those *specific patients*, rather than an acceleration of the entire regulatory review system that is contrary to the interests of public health by slackening checks on safety and efficacy generally. Sometimes pharmaceutical companies refuse to co-operate with such a 'compassionate' policy because serving the small market involved is not compatible with their commercial interests – a scenario that confirms the need to distinguish industry interests even from those of patients pressing for access to drugs without a robust evidence-base of efficacy. In other cases, patient groups may press for early general market approval of a drug, whose benefit-risk ratio is unlikely to be positive because, for the (vast) majority of patients on trials, the risks outweighed the benefits. If, in this circumstance, there is no way of predicting which patients (beyond the trial) could benefit from the drug, then the patient groups would be acting against the interests of the patients *and* public health. This is because patients who take such a drug are more likely to suffer than benefit, and future patients in this, and other therapeutic fields (public health) would lose out as lower regulatory demands (of drug efficacy, as well as safety) for marketing approval come to be accepted.

7 It is not in the interests of public health or patients, in general, for the regulatory system to increase the risk-benefit ratio of the drugs approved on to the market, even if this is done, in part, as a response to the demands of some patient groups. It is, however, in the commercial interests of the industry for drug approvals to be accelerated, even if that increases the risk-benefit ratio of new drugs. Hence, insofar as regulators respond to the demands by manufacturers and some patient groups to accelerate drug approvals in ways that are inconsistent with the scientific standards of safety and efficacy established by regulators themselves, then that response is biased in favour of industry interests and away from the interests of patients and public health.

8   Thus, inconsistencies in (industrial and regulatory) scientific knowledge-claims *are necessary*, though not sufficient, to impute the operation of bias. It might be suggested that a consistent narrative of knowledge-claims about drug safety or efficacy from a pharmaceutical company or regulatory agency could also be biased. Such a suggestion should be rejected because it renders the concept of 'bias' analytically weak, if not dysfunctional, and it seems to be premised on a confusion between objectivity and truth-value, on the one hand, and 'interest-neutrality', on the other. If a narrative of knowledge-claims is consistent, then it does not become biased merely because it is expressed by an interest group (*e.g.* a pharmaceutical company). Rather, it is an expression of knowledge-claims, undoubtedly influenced by interests, but *internally valid and unbiased*. Of course, that narrative might be shown to be biased by reference to *other* evidence, knowledge or narratives with which it is inconsistent. In that instance, however, the demonstration of bias crucially depends on, though is not established by, the identification of that inconsistency.

9   The FDA's classification system of 'priority' and 'standard' review is a less discriminating system than the (A-E) five-category classification used by the agency in the 1970s and 1980s. Compared with the earlier system, the 'priority' classification camouflages differences between new drugs of major therapeutic value and those of barely modest therapeutic significance.

References

Abraham, J. (1993) Scientific standards and institutional interests, *Social Studies of Science*, 23, 387–444.

Abraham, J. (1994) Bias in science and medical knowledge, *Sociology*, 28, 717–36.

Abraham, J. (1995a) *Science, politics and the pharmaceutical industry*. London: UCL Press.

Abraham, J. (1995b) The production and reception of scientific papers in the academic-industrial complex, *British Journal of Sociology*, 46, 167–90.

Abraham, J. (2007) From evidence to theory – neo-liberal corporate bias as a framework for understanding UK pharmaceuticals regulation, *Social Theory and Health*, 5, 161–75.

Abraham, J. and Davis, C. (2005a) A comparative analysis of drug safety withdrawals in the UK and the US (1971–1992), *Social Science and Medicine*, 61, 881–92.

Abraham, J. and Davis, C. (2005b) Risking public safety, *Health, Risk and Society*, 7, 379–95.

Abraham, J. and Davis, C. (2006) Testing times: the emergence of the Practolol disaster and its challenge to British drug regulation in the modern period, *Social History of Medicine*, 19, 127–47.

Abraham, J. and Davis, C. (2007a) Deficits, expectations and paradigms in British and American drug safety assessments, *Science, Technology and Human Values*, 32, 399–431.

Abraham, J. and Davis, C. (2007b) Interpellative sociology of pharmaceuticals, *Technology Analysis and Strategic Management*, 19, 387–402.

Abraham, J. and Lewis, G. (1999) Harmonising and competing for medicines regulation, *Social Science and Medicine*, 48, 1655–67.

Abraham, J. and Lewis, G. (2000) *Regulating Medicines in Europe*. London: Routledge.

Abraham, J. and Lewis, G. (2002) Citizenship, medical expertise and the capitalist regulatory state, *Sociology*, 36, 67–88.

Abraham, J. and Reed, T. (2001) Trading risks for markets, *Health, Risk and Society*, 3, 113–28.

Abraham, J. and Reed, T. (2002) Progress, innovation and regulatory science, *Social Studies of Science*, 32, 337–69.

Abraham, J. and Reed, T. (2003) Reshaping the carcinogenic risk assessment of medicines, *Social Science and Medicine*, 57, 195–204.

Abraham, J. and Sheppard, J. (1997) Democracy, technocracy and the secret state of medicines control, *Science, Technology and Human Values*, 22, 139–67.

Abraham, J. and Sheppard, J. (1999a) *The Therapeutic Nightmare*. London: Earthscan.

Abraham, J. and Sheppard, J. (1999b) Complacent and conflicting scientific expertise in British and American drug regulation, *Social Studies of Science*, 29, 803–44.

Adam, B., Beck, U. and Loon, J. van (2000) *The Risk Society and Beyond*. London: Sage.

Anon. (1989) US FDA/NCI reconcile differences, *Scrip* 1450, 20.

Barkan, I.D. (1985) Industry invites regulation, *American Journal of Public Health*, 75, 18–26.

Bernstein, M. (1955) *Regulating Business by Independent Commission*. New Jersey: Princeton U.P.

Bloor, D. (1973) Wittgenstein and Mannheim on the sociology of mathematics, *Studies in the History and Philosophy of Science*, 4, 173–91.

Bogard, W. (1990) Closing down the social, *Sociological Theory*, 8, 1–15.

Boreus, K. (1997) The shift to the right, *European Journal of Political Research*, 31, 257–86.

Braithwaite, J. (1984) *Corporate Crime in the Pharmaceutical Industry*. London: Routledge.

Carpenter, D.P. (2004) The political economy of FDA drug review, *Health Affairs*, 23, 52–63.

Cawson, A. (1986) *Corporatism and Political Theory*. Oxford: Basil Blackwell.

Centre for Medicines Research (2005) Innovation on the wane? *Latest News*. Available at http://www.cmr.org

Chetley, A. (1990) *A Healthy Business? World Health and the Pharmaceutical Industry*. London: Zed Books.

Collier, J. (1989) *The Health Conspiracy*. London: Century.

Collins, H.M. (1981) Stages in the empirical programme of relativism, *Social Studies of Science*, 11, 4–11.

Collins, H.M. (1995) Science studies and machine intelligence. In Jasanoff, S., Markle, G.E., Peterson, J.C. and Pinch, T. (eds) *Handbook of Science and Technology Studies*. Thousand Oaks, CA: Sage.

Collins, H.M. and Yearley, S. (1992) Epistemological chicken. In Pickering, A. (ed.) *Science as Practice and Culture*. Chicago: Chicago University Press.

Daemmrich, A. and Krucken, G. (2000) Risk versus risk, *Science as Culture*, 9, 505–34.

Dews, P. (1987) *Logics of Disintegration*. London: Verso.

Gabe, J. and Bury, M. (1988) Tranquillisers as a social problem, *Sociological Review*, 36, 320–52.

Halliday, R.G., Drasdo, A.L., Lumley, C.E. and Walker, S.R. (1997) The allocation of Resources for R and D in the world's leading pharmaceutical companies, *R and D Management*, 27, 61–65.

Hancher, L. and Moran, M. (1989) *Capitalism, Culture and Economic Regulation*. Oxford: Clarendon.

Hayek, F.A. (1967) *Studies in Philosophy, Politics and Economics*. London: Routledge and Kegan Paul.

Hilts, P.J. (2003) *Protecting America's Health*. New York: Knopf.

House of Commons (2005) Inquiry into the Influence of the Pharmaceutical Industry, Health Select Committee Hearing, 20 January, Evidence, 354–56.

IFPMA (1998) A brief history of ICH. In *ICH: Past and Future*. Geneva: IFPMA.

IFPMA (2000) *The Value and Benefits of ICH to Industry*. Geneva: IFPMA.

Irwin, A. (2001) *Sociology and the Environment*. Cambridge: Polity.

Kaitin, K.I. and Di Masi, J. (2000) Measuring the pace of new drug development in the user fee era, *Drug Information Journal*, 24, 673–80.

Kessler, D.A., Hass, A.E., Feiden, K.L., Lumpkin, M. and Temple, R. (1996) Approval of new drugs in the US, *Journal of the American Medical Association*, 276, 1826–31.

Knorr-Cetina, K.D. and Mulkay, M. (1983) Introduction: emerging principles in social studies of science. In Knorr-Cetina, K.D. and Mulkay, M. (eds) *Science Observed*. London: Sage.

McIntyre, A. (1999) *Key Issues in the Pharmaceutical Industry*. Chichester: John Wiley and Sons.

Medawar, C. (1979) *Insult or Injury? An Enquiry into the Promotion of Drug Products in the Third World*. London: Social Audit.

Mitnick, B.M. (1980) *The Political Economy of Regulation*. New York: Columbia University Press.

Owen, B. amd Braetigam, R. (1978) *The Regulation Game*. Cambridge: Ballinger.

Potter, J. (1996) *Representing Reality*. London: Sage.

Rappert, B. (2007) On the Mid Range, *Science, Technology and Human Values*, 32, 693–712.

Schwarz, M. and Thompson, M. (1990) *Divided We Stand*. London: Harvester.

Stieb, E.W. (1966) *Drug Adulteration*. Madison: University of Wisconsin Press.

Tansey, I.P., Armstrong, N.A. and Walker, S.R. (1994) Trends in pharmaceutical innovation, *Journal of Pharmaceutical Medicine*, 4, 81–5.

Van Zwanenberg, P. and Millstone, E. (2000) Beyond skeptical relativism, *Science, Technology and Human Values*, 25, 259–82.

Woolgar, S. (1981) Interests and explanation in the social study of science, *Social Studies of Science*, 11, 365–94.

Woolgar, S. (1988) *Science: the Very Idea*. London: Tavistock.

6

Sex, drugs, and politics: the HPV vaccine for cervical cancer

Monica J. Casper and Laura M. Carpenter

Introduction

A key tenet of social studies of science is that technologies are politicised (Bijker, Hughes and Pinch 1987). Social relations of sex/gender, in particular, may shape their development, and assumptions about men and women, masculinity and femininity, infuse sociotechnical objects. Although this is true for many technologies, these dynamics are especially visible in sexual and reproductive health technologies. Recent investigations (*e.g.* Loe 2006) show not only that these technologies are permeated with meanings of sex/gender, but also that their use impacts on social relations, both exposing politics of gender and sexuality and transforming practices.

This chapter examines the emergence and contested use of a new gendered technology: the human papillomavirus (HPV) vaccine for cervical cancer (CC). Gardasil, manufactured by pharmaceutical giant Merck and Co. Inc. (hereafter, Merck), was approved by the United States Food and Drug Administration (FDA) in 2006; by year's end, sales totalled $235 million. A second vaccine, Cervarix, produced by GlaxoSmithKline (hereafter, GSK), is scheduled for market in 2008. Both vaccines are reported to be almost completely effective in preventing development of 70 per cent of cervical abnormalities.

The vaccine has many enthusiasts: women's health advocates, clinicians, public health officials, women at risk, and industry. Yet it has become embroiled in intense controversy. Some US conservatives dubbed it 'the promiscuity vaccine' (Gibbs 2006), while anti-vaccinationists targeted mandatory vaccine legislation and safety and efficacy. As with other sexualised technologies (*e.g.* Viagra, male contraception), the HPV vaccine cannot be understood outside gender relations and attendant cultural politics. Here, we offer a sociological analysis of this new pharmaceutical and the ways in which it both reveals and animates the social relations of sexuality and gender.

Pharmacologies of containment

In examining the HPV vaccine as a gendered pharmaceutical technology, we are guided by the work of scholars who investigate the 'ethics, markets, [and] practices' of 'Big Pharma' (Petryna, Lakoff and Kleinman 2006). Pharmaceuticals offer an ideal opportunity to study the relationship between symbols and political economy. Van der Geest *et al.* (1996) position drugs as commodities with distinctive biographies. '[A] "biography" of pharmaceuticals is a metaphor . . . people give these substances a history. As powerful technical devices and status symbols, medicines acquire a status and force in society' (1996: 156). Following the transactions of these objects reveals a biographical order – and a gendered technical order – to their social life.

Pharmaceuticals may profoundly *transform* social relations, thus rendering useful a consideration of politics – understood as various struggles shaped by power and its operations. In Van der Geest *et al.*'s biographical approach, politics is framed simply as the 'context' for the pharmaceutical lifecourse. In our view, politics is more fundamental, implicated in every stage of pharmaceuticals' biographical lives (production and marketing, prescription, distribution, use, efficacy). Politics shape the ways drugs are produced, used, and so forth; but drugs may also instigate political struggles, and, potentially, social change, over their lifecourses, as well as embodying extant conflicts.

Technologies such as the HPV vaccine represent a specific kind of pharmaceutical, geared not towards therapy per se (as, for example, analgesics are), but rather, toward *containment* (Bashford and Hooker 2001). Because vaccines target infectious diseases, they are immediately implicated in the politics of contagion, which elicits a sense of danger, risk, invasion, and vulnerability. Contagion is *always* about contact, and frequently invokes notions of transmission – because it is about the intimacies shared among people – and as such requires 'the establishment of cordons sanitaire in one form or another, the drawing of lines and zones of hygiene' (Bashford and Hooker 2001: 9). These demarcations are formed within particular social, political, economic, and geographic contexts, from which they take their meanings.

The HPV vaccine prevents cervical cancer by controlling an infectious agent; thus, strategies of containment are incorporated into its design and function. It is, in our view, a pharmaceutical cordon sanitaire. And yet, it is currently a dubious one, particularly in the US. While the vaccine's technical efficacy is considerable (some questions about its overall and long-term efficacy remain (Sawaya and Smith-McCune 2007)), its social and cultural efficacy are at issue in the controversy surrounding its distribution and use – the biographical stages upon which we focus here. The HPV vaccine embodies the 'dream of hygienic containment' (Bashford and Hooker 2001), and consequently, it has activated deep social and cultural cleavages related to sexuality, gender, and health care. Invoking notions of danger and risk, the HPV vaccine is poised to transform bodies, institutions, and practices. In exposing the interrelated social processes of contagion and containment, we offer a sociological account of how a pharmaceutical technology may be deeply, irrevocably intimate.

Cervical cancer and HPV

The cervix comprises the lower part of the uterus and is divided from the upper uterus and vagina by the os (Singer and Jordan 2006). It is covered by two layers of epithelia: an inner basal columnar epithelium and a thin outer tissue layer made of flat, irregularly shaped squamous cells. The cervical epithelium undergoes many changes, beginning during fetal life and continuing until menopause; 'the result is a dynamic epithelium of varied morphology' (2006: 35). Physiological dynamism renders the cervix susceptible to malignancies.

Cervical cancer is a common disease affecting only women. While there has long been confusion surrounding CC classification systems (Clarke and Casper 1996) it is now understood that initial stages of CC, known as squamous cell carcinomas, account for about 80 per cent of all invasive cases. The World Health Organization (WHO) recognises early CC as cervical intraepithelial neoplasia (CIN) or squamous intraepithelial lesion (SIL) (Koushik and Franco 2006). CIN and SIL are typically asymptomatic, and are detected only through screening technologies (Casper and Clarke 1998). Untreated precursors can develop into carcinoma, hence prevention is critical to reduced incidence.

Worldwide, approximately 493,000 new cases of CC are diagnosed annually (Koushik and Franco 2006). Cervical cancer represents 10 per cent of all female cancers, is eighth among cancer sites, and in women is second only to breast cancer. Of the 225,000 annual deaths from CC, 80–85 per cent are in developing countries (Dailard 2006), reflecting limited access to health care and preventive technologies. Comparatively, in the US, where preventive screening is routine for most women, CC is relatively rare. In 2006, there were 10,000 cases resulting in 3,700 deaths. Yet American mortality and morbidity are stratified by race/ethnicity and socioeconomic status (Singh *et al.* 2004).

Cervical cancer was long considered to be just that, a cancer, and prevention and treatment proceeded accordingly. A major etiological shift occurred in the 1990s, and CC is now widely understood to be a sexually transmitted infection (STI), with HPV acknowledged as the causal agent (Koushik and Franco 2006). The connection was clearly established when German researchers isolated and cloned a new type of HPV taken from a cervical biopsy (Durst *et al.* 1983). Subsequent studies 'demonstrated that HPV infection results in virtually all diagnosed cases of cervical cancer and preinvasive cytopathologic precursors' (Grimes 2006: 150).

The science and politics of cancer have been challenged and reconfigured by virology – and vice versa. A key feature of this transformation is the difficulty of determining what HPV is, virologically, and who gets it, epidemiologically. Over 100 types of HPV have been identified to date, 30 of them transmissible via sex, making HPV the most common STI in the world.[1] Yet while some HPV types develop into CC, many do not (Lowy and Schiller 2006). Implications of this are manifold: on the one hand, recognition of the link prompted development of the prophylactic vaccine, while on the other hand, there is considerable uncertainty among clinicians, health officials, and the public about what HPV is, how to prevent it, and its relationship to CC.

The HPV vaccine

Gardasil and Cervarix are noninfectious, recombinant vaccines; they stimulate an immune response but cannot cause HPV because they are made with proteins that contain only part of the virus (Wheeler 2007). Both target HPV-16 and HPV-18, which together account for about 70 per cent of cervical cancers. Gardasil additionally targets HPV-6 and HPV-11, which produce 90 per cent of genital warts. Cervarix is formulated with AS04, an adjuvant intended to strengthen and prolong immune system response (GlaxoSmithKline 2007). Clinical trials indicate that Cervarix may also protect against HPV-45 and HPV-31, the third and fourth most common cancer-causing strains (Harper *et al.* 2006).

Both vaccines are administered by injection in three doses, Gardasil at 0, 2 and 6 months, and Cervarix at 0, 1 and 6 months. A three-shot course of Gardasil costs about US$360, and Cervarix is expected to be comparably priced. Side effects are generally minor: localised itching and swelling, and systemic dizziness, fever, and nausea (Wheeler 2007). As of May 2007, 136 'serious adverse reactions' to Gardasil had been recorded, including seizures, Guillain-Barre Syndrome, miscarriages or fetal abnormalities, and three deaths (which the US Centers for Disease Control (CDC), FDA, and Merck claim were unrelated to the vaccine) (Carreyrou 2007).

Young women are the target population for two reasons. First, Merck's trials found stronger immunological response in girls aged 10–15 than in women aged 16–23 (Dailard 2006). Secondly, the vaccine is more efficacious among women who have not yet had sex (Kaiser Family Foundation 2007). One study found that Gardasil was 99 per cent effective in preventing cervical cancer and pre-cancerous lesions in women who had never had (vaginal) sex but only 44 per cent effective in sexually-experienced women, who potentially had been exposed to HPV (Ault *et al.* 2007). Gardasil is being tested on men who could benefit from the vaccine's protection against genital warts (CDC 2006).

Cervarix began the FDA approval process in March 2007. But where Gardasil was granted a fast-track review,[2] the FDA declined to do the same for Cervarix, probably because of safety concerns about GSK's fast-tracked diabetes drug, Avandia (Wardell 2007). If the standard 10-month review is successful, Cervarix should hit the US market in 2008. Phase III trial data indicate 'demonstrated antibody response against HPV-16 and HPV-18' among 100 per cent of women aged 15–55 at one and six months after completing the vaccination course (Schwarz and Dubin 2006).

Merck and GSK stand to profit considerably. If the vaccine becomes routine for teenage girls, and if it is incorporated into government-funded vaccination programmes, analysts predict annual US sales of $3.2 billion (Allen 2007). Notably, the success of Gardasil would benefit not only Merck, but also its competitor, as GSK receives royalties on Gardasil sales due to a 2005 settlement agreement over patents (Lawler 2007). Both companies face revenue losses following research linking blockbuster drugs Vioxx (Merck) and Avandia (GSK) to increased health risks and the release of best-selling medications to generic competition (Capell 2004). The HPV vaccine thus takes part in the broader economic relations of Big Pharma.

Merck publicly aborted its campaign for mandatory vaccination following the February 2007 revelation that Women in Government, an organisation which had spearheaded state-by-state lobbying in support of vaccine mandates for adolescent girls, received money from Merck (Allen 2007). Additional ethical concerns stemmed from the presence of two former Merck employees on the FDA committee that approved Gardasil.

'Calling the shots': HPV vaccine and health-care politics

The HPV vaccine enters into an existing set of public health and clinical arrangements, which vary by geography, governance, and financing structure. Given the principal locus of controversy, we focus on the vaccine's impact on US health care, a fragmented, multi-payer, for-profit system. Structural conditions contribute to controversy surrounding the vaccine. Capital-intensive, private, technology-driven health care has led to an impoverished public health infrastructure (Boylan 2006), and in 2006 the number of uninsured Americans was at an all-time high of 46.6 million, nine million of whom were children.[3]

Patient-provider relations
Clinicians are central to the distribution of the HPV vaccine: they administer it to patients on three occasions. Positioned to make important decisions about girls and women for whom the vaccine is indicated, clinicians are key figures in the cultural politics surrounding the vaccine's acceptance and use, including its incorporation into women's routine preventive health care. Thus, the vaccine reveals gendered aspects of the doctor-patient relationship while creating new categories of patients and new pathways to medicalisation of girls' bodies.

Raley and colleagues (2004) found that the variable most influencing a gynecologist's decision to recommend the HPV vaccine was the professional organisation's position. This is noteworthy, given that the American College of Obstetricians and Gynecologists (ACOG) strongly supports the HPV vaccine. Describing it as 'a significant development in women's health and the fight against cancer', President Douglas W. Laube declared, 'Obstetrician-gynecologists should be proactive in educating our patients . . . so that as many women as possible are able to take advantage of this medical milestone' (ACOG 2006). The Society for Adolescent Medicine (SAM) holds a similar view, endorsing the US Advisory Committee on Immunization Practices' (ACIP) recommendation as well as advocating coverage by third-party payers and public funds.

Yet some practitioners oppose widespread HPV vaccination on grounds of safety and efficacy. Lowndes and Gill (2005) note 'important questions need answering before a program of HPV vaccination can be introduced' (2005: 916), including the proportion of cervical cancer cases attributable to HPV in various regions/countries, the fraction of CC prevented by vaccination, the need for booster vaccinations, the vaccine's impact on screening programmes, and cost effectiveness. Expressing concern that data on Gardasil's safety and efficacy have come from small groups of women, Sawaya and Smith-McCune (2007) assert 'while the trials are ongoing, mandatory vaccination is premature'.

Practitioners may also oppose HPV vaccination on moral grounds. Clinicians' beliefs about sexuality and adolescence may influence their acceptance of the vaccine, and consequently their recommendations to patients. In one survey, 63 per cent of physicians 'said it would be ethical for morally conflicted doctors to "plainly" explain their objections to their patients' and only 86 per cent felt obliged to present all medical options (Curlin *et al.* 2007). Mays and Zimet (2004) found nurse practitioners were reluctant to vaccinate younger adolescents for STIs, especially since they were lacking endorsement from the American Academy of Pediatrics (AAP). Thus, many women at risk for CC may be treated by physicians who do not believe they must disclose information about medical options they personally find objectionable.

Emergent health-care markets
New drugs may reorder or forge new health-care practices and markets. The target population for the HPV vaccine – girls and young women – is demographically appropriate for provision of health care within adolescent medicine, thus the HPV vaccine is positioned to reshape and advance that field. Scientific advances in endocrinology and gynecology, along with concerns about increased mortality among adolescents, contributed to the development, over a century, of a distinct sub-specialty focused on teenagers and their needs (Alderman *et al.* 2003): 'The most notable change . . . was the shift from the traditional role of providing anticipatory guidance to parents toward a reduction of risk-taking behaviors aimed directly at the adolescent' (2003: 137).

The vaccine is currently administered by a diverse group of gynecologists, pediatricians, general practitioners, and family physicians, yet already, clinicians recognise the ways in which the HPV vaccine could serve as the basis for co-ordinating and expanding adolescent health care – an important change in the social organisation of medicine. In 1996, the Advisory Committee on Immunization Practices joined with other groups to identify ages 11–12 as the optimal period for adolescent immunisations. The US Childhood and Adolescent Immunization Schedule recommends that every 11–12-year-old receive two vaccines (one for meningitis and the other a combined tetanus-diphtheria-whooping cough booster) and be 'caught-up' on other shots. The HPV vaccine has been added to this schedule. Zimet (2005: S22) suggests that 'the recent and future emergence of multiple vaccines . . . for preadolescents and adolescents provides us with a unique opportunity to provide a valuable package of preventive interventions for adolescents'.

With their history of addressing clinical and social concerns of teenagers, adolescent health-care providers are situated to promote their own professional interests alongside the HPV vaccine – effectively shifting social practices in response to the pharmaceutical's advent.

Cervical cancer screening
Although some commentators have enthusiastically greeted the HPV vaccine, many are more cautious. As Jacob *et al.* (2005: 638) argue, 'widespread vaccination against HPV . . . [is] many years away' and 'any vaccine developed in the near term is unlikely to be effective

against all HPV types'. Consequently, some experts worry that the pharmaceutical will alter screening practices prematurely. The American College of Obstetricians and Gynecologists (2006) emphasises that 'current cervical cytology screening recommendations remain unchanged and should be followed regardless of vaccination status'. The most effective approach will probably be a combination of vaccination and screening, complicated by health disparities and stratified access to prevention.

Nazeer (2006: 431) calls for 'intensify[ing] efforts at [the] international and national level to increase awareness . . . [of] cervical cancer screening programs'. In resource-poor settings locally and especially globally, there is limited to no infrastructure for public health screening. Morbidity and mortality rates are high precisely because such prevention is lacking, as is sufficient treatment (WHO 2006). The Alliance for Cervical Cancer Prevention works to enhance screening in the developing world.

The HPV vaccine illuminates these disparities, providing impetus for changes in social practice. In conjunction with advocating access to the vaccine, public health officials and non-governmental organizations may push for expanded and improved screening programmes and work to ensure the vaccine is not 'beyond the reach of many women in the developing world' (WHO 2006) – or locally.

Vaccination practices
Colgrove (2006) documents the politicised nature of vaccination in the US. At the heart of controversies are the twin threats of risk and coercion, which invoke fears about state power vis-à-vis the individual, parental rights, violations of children's bodies, liberty versus the common good, and the intrusive reach of science and medicine. Colgrove argues, 'because the benefit vaccination offers – the absence of disease – is a "negative" or unapparent one, its risks, though rare, seem more salient . . . the invocation of a certain number of illnesses or deaths that did not occur has much less rhetorical force when placed against numbers of vaccine adverse events, even if the latter are very few' (2006: 8). A tension between persuasion and compulsion has characterised a century of debates – with consequences for epidemiology, clinical practice, health, and public perception of pharmaceuticals.

The emergence of the HPV vaccine stimulated these tensions. Despite support for the vaccine among clinicians, youth, and parents, the issue of compulsion has ignited controversy across the US. Some states have pursued legislation mandating the vaccine for schoolchildren, while others have sought to require that health insurers operating in the state cover the vaccine or that public schools provide information about the vaccine. Almost every school mandate effort has failed (see below); however, in states like New Hampshire, a 'soft sell' approach encouraging but not requiring vaccination has created a demand for the vaccine so huge it cannot be satisfied (National Conference of State Legislatures (NCSL) 2007).

At issue in current debates about mandatory school vaccination, as historically, are parental rights and the state's reach (Colgrove 2006). Certain critics see public health information, not government mandates, as a more optimal way to encourage vaccination. Some opponents also argue that school vaccination mandates interfere with abstinence-focused sex education policies. Across the US, in the backlash against compulsion, parents are asserting their rights to make decisions about not only their children's health care, but also their sexual and reproductive health education.

Debates about mandatory vaccination are about more than parental rights. In the conservative climate of the US the battle cry of 'family values' can quash public debate. Struggles over mandatory legislation allow parents and others to pay lip service to the utility of the HPV vaccine, while making access difficult for the women who most need it. Although ACIP's recommendation guarantees access for uninsured girls through the federal Vaccines for Children program, without school mandates, many parents (regardless of insurance status) may decline to vaccinate their daughters, leaving the girls at risk for HPV and cervical cancer.

Mandates' economic benefits to individuals are often overlooked. If vaccines are required for schoolchildren and are included in government schedules, then third-party payers will be more likely to reimburse for vaccination, and public payers must ensure widespread coverage. This translates into increased access for low-income girls and women without health insurance – precisely those most at risk for developing cervical cancer. Insurance mandates likewise increase access to the vaccine. Legislative mandates for schoolchildren and insurance companies may substantially reduce gaps in access to the HPV vaccine – although existing gaps in screening will remain.

'Sending the wrong message': HPV vaccine and sexual politics

Longstanding tensions among different perspectives on sexual activity reached unprecedented levels in late 20th century America (Seidman 1991). Although sex before marriage was not uncommon before World War II (despite ideals valuing premarital virginity), postwar economic prosperity, combined with the Baby Boom, had by the late 1960s produced a heterosexual youth culture that *openly* rejected premarital chastity, and had sex with partners they had no expectations of marrying (D'Emilio and Freedman 1988). These changes affected young women especially, as the feminist movement's demand for equality and development of birth control enhanced their ability and desire to breach tradition.

Starting in the mid-1970s, the Christian Right launched a series of crusades intended to reverse the growing 'permissiveness' of US sexual culture (Irvine 2002). Aiming at such targets as legalised abortion, gay rights, and an 'epidemic' of teen pregnancy, they achieved considerable success. A chief battle site has been sex education policy. Although the vast majority of US adults approve of school-based *comprehensive* sex education programmes, moral conservatives have succeeded in making *abstinence-only* curricula the law of the land (Dailard 2001). Federal funding for sex education, which few states can afford to refuse, requires recipients to teach that sexual abstinence until marriage 'is the only certain way to avoid out-of-wedlock pregnancy, sexually transmitted diseases, and other associated health problems' (Advocates for Youth and SIECUS 2001). Such curricula do not result in delayed first intercourse, lower rates of STIs, or prevent teen pregnancy (Kirby 2002) and medical organisations oppose them. Yet, the proportion of US public school districts offering comprehensive sex education shrank significantly over the 1980s and 1990s, while the proportion teaching abstinence-only curricula increased (Dailard 2001).

Moral conservatives' victories largely curbed, rather than reversed, the liberalising tendencies of previous decades. The average age at first (hetero)sex plateaued around 1990 and rose slightly from 1995 to 2002, especially among men (Risman and Schwartz 2002). Few American teenagers (about 14% in 2002) have engaged in vaginal sex before age 15, although over 60 per cent of 17-year-olds have (Abma *et al.* 2004). It is of particular relevance to the HPV vaccine that about half of sexually active women aged 19–21 report having had four or more sexual partners (Wheeler 2007), and African Americans, the racial/ethnic group most at risk for cervical cancer, become sexually active at earlier ages than Whites (Upchurch *et al.* 1998).

Gender, youth, and sexuality

Beliefs that young women are sexually endangered and in need of protection – yet are also threatening to society if uncontrolled, and therefore (ironically) responsible for regulating sexual activity – have endured. These convictions derive in part from age-old efforts to control human reproduction, which disproportionately target women because pregnancy makes their role in reproduction more visible than men's, and to enjoin post-pubertal youth to postpone childbearing until they are 'ready' according to social norms (Nathanson 1991).

For over a century, popular and scientific opinion has held that (White, middle-class) women are inherently less sexual than men, as well as generally more fragile and in need of protection (Nathanson 1991). These gendered and racialised beliefs have fostered a sexual double standard: (some) women are to be protected, while (some) men are encouraged to sow wild oats (D'Emilio and Freedman 1988). Ever since the sexual 'revolution' of the 1960s, women are expected to reserve sex for love, while casual sex is acceptable for men (Rubin 1990).

The idea that children are sexually innocent, especially before puberty, is age old, as is the conviction that youth are highly suggestible, easily 'infected' by all manner of potentially undesirable behaviours (Levine 2002). Believing that sexual activity is inherently dangerous to youth and fearing that youth will mimic the sexual behaviours to which they are exposed, parents, politicians, and policymakers have sought to curb young people's activities by controlling access to sexual information in mass media and schools.[4] A majority of US adults believe it is wrong for adolescents, especially those younger than 16, to be sexually active, though only a minority disapprove of premarital sex per se (Widmer et al. 1998).

Cultural assumptions about youth and gender are not without critics from the Left, notably pro-sex feminists and progressive sex educators, and from the Right, especially proponents of premarital chastity for women and men. Nor are they borne out by American adolescents' actual behaviour. But they do powerfully affect public policy and social practices around the HPV vaccine.

Inflammation and contention

Initially, many public health institutions, medical associations, and state governments – eager to harness a new technology in their efforts to protect young women – embraced the HPV vaccine. Within weeks of FDA approval of Gardasil, ACIP unanimously approved a provisional recommendation that all girls aged 11–12 receive the vaccine. This was formalised in January 2007, with inclusion of the HPV vaccine in the CDC's Child and Adolescent Vaccination Schedule. Leading medical associations endorsed the recommendations.

Feminist and progressive sex education organisations heralded the vaccine as a pharmaceutical lifesaver, a sentiment echoed in the popular press. Planned Parenthood Federation of America (PPFA) urged ACIP to make 'access to the vaccine . . . a public health priority', and the National Organization for Women (NOW) 'congratulate[d] the US [FDA] for approving a vaccine that could save hundreds of thousands of women from cancer-causing strains of [HPV]'. Newspaper editorials pronounced benefits of the vaccine as 'too great to ignore' and – cognisant of a key conservative objection – noted that no studies had linked vaccination to increased sexual activity, 'any more than there is evidence that giving people tetanus shots encourages them to step on rusty nails' (Los Angeles Times 2006).

In September 2006, Michigan became the first state to introduce legislation to require, fund, and/or educate the public about the vaccine (NCSL 2007). By January 2007, 11 states were considering similar measures; by late February, that number had jumped to 20. Yet by May 2007, of the 24 states plus the District of Columbia that introduced mandatory vaccination bills, only Virginia had enacted a law. Conservative committee members prevented bills from coming to full-chamber debates or votes in several states and sponsors withdrew bills from consideration even in liberal stalwarts (NCSL 2007). In May 2007, the Arizona legislature approved a bill *prohibiting* the state's health department from requiring the vaccine. Nationally, a Republican congressman introduced the *Parental Right to Decide Protection Act*, meant to prohibit the use of federal monies to establish mandatory HPV vaccination programmes.

Failure of so many pro-vaccine initiatives was due to moral conservatives' vigorous opposition, in co-operation with parental rights groups and vaccination opponents. Conservatives' reservations about vaccinating preteen girls centre on the concern that doing so 'is going to sabotage our abstinence message', which stresses negative consequences (Stein 2005). In particular, they cite 'disinhibition' effects, whereby vaccinated individuals are thought to eschew precautions because they (falsely) believe themselves to be protected from harm. Conservatives endeavour to protect youth and women from physical *and moral* harm by containing their sexuality.

Initially, flagship groups Family Research Council (FRC) and Focus on the Family (FOF) appeared poised to reject the vaccine altogether (Stein 2005). They quickly moderated their stance, apparently in response to Merck's reassurances that there was 'no evidence for any increase in sexual disinhibition in connection with the vaccine' (FRC 2007), and the fact that a former FOF medical analyst served on ACIP while the vaccine was under consideration. CDC also countered claims about disinhibition effects, noting that other fear factors (*e.g.*, HIV, pregnancy) would remain in effect.

Some conservatives pursued *scientific* challenges. The organisation Judicial Watch used the *Freedom of Information Act* to obtain data on three vaccine-related deaths, which, when widely publicised, fanned concerns about safety (Carreyrou 2007). At the time of writing, however, most conservative organisations acknowledge that the vaccine reduces risk of cervical cancer and 'suppor[t] routine but not mandatory vaccination against HPV for adolescent females' (Medical Institute for Sexual Health), even as their policy statements insist that 'the HPV vaccine does not, in any circumstance, negate or substitute God's plan for sexuality, which is sexual abstinence until marriage and sexual faithfulness within marriage' (FOF 2006). Such claims suggest that, safety arguments notwithstanding, moral concerns are paramount for social conservatives.

Curiously, the statement, 'Clarification of 2005 Family Research Council Media Remarks on HPV Vaccine', affirming the organisation's support for the vaccine since late 2005, was issued in February 2007, suggesting that FRC felt compelled to respond to critics who accused it of promoting abstinence over cancer prevention. With the vaccine threatening their claim that 'only abstinence can solve sex-related ills', conservatives aimed to regain the upper hand in the sex wars by shifting the terms of the debate from *providing* the vaccine (acceptable) to *mandating* the vaccine (unacceptable) – even as they continued to insist that abstinence offers the best protection.

Left-of-centre organisations were swift to counter moral conservatives. *Nation* columnist Katha Pollitt (2005) wrote: 'With HPV potentially eliminated, the antisex brigade will lose a [trump] card . . . unless it can persuade parents that vaccinating their daughters will turn them into tramps, and that sex today is worse than cancer tomorrow'. NOW roundly criticised conservatives for 'show[ing] that they are more concerned with women's chastity than their health' (Richert 2005), and Planned Parenthood Federation of America assistant director Cantu Hinojosa said of the legislative setbacks, 'It's really a shame that politics and ideology are getting in the way of saving lives'.

In short, sexual progressives responded to the HPV debate as in previous skirmishes, by denouncing sex education based on fear. They also seemed to hope that the link between HPV and CC would push debate to a new level, forcing previously silent moderates to realise how extreme and dangerous the moral conservative position was (on silent moderates, see Irvine 2002).

These debates have affected public opinion about the HPV vaccine, in ways likely to affect social practice. A 2003 study found that a majority of parents were in favour of the vaccine being available and that parents who believed their children were at risk for HPV were more accepting of the vaccine (Olshen 2005). By 2007, the National Poll on Children's Health found only 44 per cent of parents were in favour of mandatory HPV vaccination, compared with 68 per cent for the combined tetanus-diphtheria-pertussis (Tdap) vaccine. Study authors claimed that parents' attitudes toward mandates for the HPV vaccine were largely due to concerns about vaccine safety, *not* 'promiscuity', suggesting a disjuncture between moral conservatives and American parents overall (like that regarding sex education). However, parents with children under six were more likely to support a vaccine mandate than parents with children aged 6 to 17 – suggesting that parental attitudes may shift as children approach sexual maturity (*Medical News Today* 2007). Despite parents' stated concern with safety, then, unease about moral issues appears to play a critical role.

On balance, the HPV vaccine controversy has reinforced prevailing understandings of women as responsible for controlling sexual activity and reproduction – *and* as sexually innocent and endangered. Yet a significant threat to young women – unwanted sex and abuse – is surprisingly absent from current debates; moral conservatives seem not to have recognised the need to protect 'presexual' girls from assailant-transmitted HPV.

Conclusions

Containment technologies like the HPV vaccine may prevent infection, but they do not contain politics, as our analysis demonstrates. Pharmaceutical biographies, far from simply unfolding against a political background, interact with and alter the political and cultural landscape – (re)shaping the pharmaceutical's lifecourse in turn. Epistemological and practical confusion surrounding CC and HPV, and the vaccine targeting them, contribute to political struggles that are sexualised and gendered. These struggles are consequential for perceptions and use of the vaccine, and for the social worlds in which it is deployed.

Yet vaccines are distinctive from other pharmaceuticals – and the HPV vaccine differs from its kin in crucial ways. All vaccines embody – and rely on – the politics of contagion and containment. But because the HPV vaccine's target is *sexually* transmitted, it provokes longstanding controversies swirling around sex, gender, and women's bodies in the US. Not surprisingly, Merck, GSK, and pro-vaccine actors frame the issue as cancer, not HPV – taking advantage of the lag in public perception of cervical cancer as an STI and suppressing the gendered dimensions of both diseases. As Nathanson (2007) demonstrates, framing risks in culturally-palatable ways is critical to the development of public health policies. Connecting the HPV vaccine to cancer rather than sexual domains *may* diminish the controversy associated with it, but whether such a diminution will occur over time remains an empirical question.

Our analysis of the HPV vaccine has revealed aspects of the social relations of sexuality, gender, and age while also showing how the technology has precipitated shifts in the organisation of health care. These shifts too are gendered. Technical innovations such as youth-targeted vaccines spur the growth and consolidation of adolescent medicine. But the specific configurations of clinical practice related to the HPV vaccine are clearly related to contested cultural understandings of young women's sexuality.

This was not the case for another vaccine targeting an STI. According to James Colgrove,[5] the vaccine against Hepatitis B did not inspire such controversy – despite expectations – because Hepatitis B is also (if rarely) transmitted through non-sexual means. The vaccine was developed in 1981, an earlier juncture in US sexual and health politics; it was more widely accepted/proven in the medical community; and it was administered in very early childhood, when the spectres of puberty and sexual activity are less haunting.

In sum, the launch of the HPV vaccine has inflamed existing US health care and sexual politics, which have, in turn, affected plans for marketing the drug (and possibly Cervarix's journey through FDA). Signifying the scale of struggles provoked by this new gendered technology, both Merck and GSK stress that they have been meeting groups 'across the political spectrum' (Stein 2005), ostensibly to enrol supporters, gain allies and minimise controversy. Clearly, a pharmaceutical's biography, just like a human's, is ever emergent and evolving.

Notes

1 See the US Centers for Disease Control and Prevention website at http://www.cdc.gov/std/hpv/.
2 See Hilts (2003) for a discussion of 'fast tracking' at the FDA.
3 Online NewsHour, 'Number of Americans without health insurance hits record high', 30 August 2006. http://www.pbs.org/newshour/bb/health/july-dec06/insurance_08-30.html
4 Research routinely fails to substantiate these fears (Advocates for Youth and SIECUS 2001).
5 Personal communication, 1 June 2007.

References

Abma, J.C., Martinez, G.M., Mosher, W.D. and Dawson, B.S. (2004) Teenagers in the United States: sexual activity, contraceptive use, and childbearing 2002, *Vital and Health Statistics*, 23, 24.

Advocates for Youth, and SIECUS (2001) *Toward a Sexually Healthy America: Roadblocks Imposed by the Federal Government's Abstinence-only-until-marriage Education Program*. New York: Advocates for Youth and SIECUS.

Alderman, E.M., Rieder, J. and Cohen, M.I. (2003) The history of adolescent medicine, *Pediatric Research*, 54, 1, 137–47.

Allen, T.J. (2007) Merck's murky dealings: HPV vaccine lobby backfires, 13 June. See http://www.corpwatch.org/article.php?id=14401

American College of Obstetricians and Gynecologists (2006) ACOG releases HPV vaccine recommendations for ob-gyns, 8 August. See www.acog.org.

Ault, K.A. for the Future II Study Group (2007) Effect of prophylactic human papillomavirus L1 virus-like-particle vaccine on risk of cervical intraepithelial neoplasia grade 2, grade 3, and adenocarcinoma in situ: a combined analysis of four randomised clinical trials, *Lancet*, 369, 1861–8.

Bashford, A. and Hooker, C. (2001) *Contagion: Historical and Cultural Studies*. London: Routledge.

Bijker, W.E., Hughes, T.P. and Pinch, T. (eds) (1987) *The Social Construction of Technological Systems: New Directions in the Sociology and History of Technology*. Cambridge: MIT Press.

Boylan, M. (ed.) (2006) *Public Health Policy and Ethics*. New York: Springer.

Capell, K. (2004) A vaccine every woman should take, *Business Week online*, 29 Nov.

Carreyrou, J. (2007) FDA data on Gardasil may fuel controversy, *Wall Street Journal*, 24 May.

Casper, M.J. and Clarke, A.E. (1998) Making the Pap smear into the 'right tool' for the job: cervical cancer screening in the USA, circa 1940–95, *Social Studies of Science*, 28, 2, 255–90.

CDC (Centers for Disease Control) (2006) *HPV Vaccine Questions and Answers*. See http://www.cdc.gov/std/hpv/STDFact-HPV-vaccine.htm#hpvvac1

Clarke, A.E. and Casper, M.J. (1996) From simple technology to complex arena: classification of Pap smears, 1917–1990, *Medical Anthropology Quarterly*, 10, 4, 601–23.

Colgrove, J. (2006) *State of Immunity: the Politics of Vaccination in Twentieth-century America*. Berkeley: University of California Press.

Curlin, F.A., Lawrence, R., Chin, M.H. and Lantos, J.D. (2007) Religion, conscience and controversial clinical practices, *New England Journal of Medicine*, 356, 6, 593–600.

Dailard, C. (2001) Sex education: politicians, parents, teachers, and teens, *The Guttmacher Report on Public Policy*, 4, 1, 9–12.

Dailard, C. (2006) The public health promise and potential pitfalls of the world's first cervical cancer vaccine, *Guttmacher Policy Review*, 9, 1, 6–9.

D'Emilio, J. and Freedman, E.B. (1988) *Intimate Matters: a History of Sexuality in America*. New York: Harper and Row.

Durst, M., Gissman, L., Ikenberg, H. and zur Hausen, H. (1983) A papillomavirus DNA from a cervical carcinoma and its prevalence in cancer biopsy samples from different geographic regions, *Proceedings of the National Academy of Science*, 80, 3812–15.

Family Research Council (2007) Clarification of 2005 Family Research Council Media Remarks on HPV Vaccine, 12 February. http://www.frc.org/get.cfm?i=LH07B02

Focus on the Family (2006) Position statement: human papillomavirus vaccines, 19 January. See www.family.org

FDA (US Food and Drug Administration) (2007) *Product Approval Information – Licensing Action: GARDASIL® Questions and Answers*. See http://www.fda.gov/cber/products/hpvmer060806qa.htm

Gibbs, N. (2006) Defusing the war over the 'promiscuity' vaccine, *Time*, 21 June.

GlaxoSmithKline (2007) *Cervarix is Approved in Australia for Females 10–45 Years Old*, 21 May. See http://www.gsk.com/ControllerServlet?appId=4&pageId=402&newsid=1037

Grimes, J.L. (2006) HPV vaccine development: a case study of prevention and politics, *Biochemistry and Molecular Biology Education*, 34, 2, 148–54.

Harper, D., Franco, E., Wheeler, C. *et al.* (2006) Sustained efficacy up to 4.5 years of a bivalent L1 virus-like particle vaccine against human papillomavirus types 16 and 18: follow-up from a randomised control trial, *Lancet*, 367, 1247–55.

Hilts, P.J. (2003) *Protecting America's Health: the FDA, Business, and One Hundred Years of Regulation*. Chapel Hill: University of North Carolina Press.

Irvine, J. (2002) *Talk about Sex: the Battles over Sex Education in the United States*. Berkeley: University of California Press.

Jacob, M., Bradley, J. and Barone, M. (2005) Human papillomavirus vaccines: what does the future hold for preventing cervical cancer in resource-poor settings through immunization programs? *Sexually Transmitted Diseases*, 32, 10, 635.

Kaiser Family Foundation (2007) Fact sheet: HPV vaccine: implementation and financing policy, January. See www.kff.org.

Kirby, D. (2002) *Do Abstinence-only Programs Delay the Initiation of Sex among Young People and Reduce Teen Pregnancy?* Washington, DC: National Campaign to Prevent Teen Pregnancy.

Koushik, A. and Franco, E.L.F. (2006) Epidemiology and the role of human papillomaviruses. In Jordan, J.A. and Singer, A. (eds) *The Cervix*. 2nd edition. Oxford: Blackwell Publishing.

Lawler, B. (2007) GlaxoSmithKline gets ready for the vaccine wars, *Motley Fool*, see www.fool.com, 13 June.

Levine, J. (2002) *Harmful to Minors: the Perils of Protecting Children from Sex*. Minneapolis: University of Minnesota Press.

Loe, M. (2006) *The Rise of Viagra: how the Little Blue Pill Changed Sex in America*. New York: NYU Press.

Los Angeles Times (2006) Los Angeles Unified School District 'Right' to offer Merck's HPV vaccine to female middle, elementary school students this fall. 18 August.

Lowndes, C.M. and Gill, O.N. (2005) Cervical cancer, human papillomavirus, and vaccination, *British Medical Journal*, 331, 915–16.

Lowy, D.R. and Schiller, J.T. (2006) Prophylactic human papillomavirus vaccine, *Journal of Clinical Investigation*, 116, 5, 1167–73.

Mays, R.M. and Zimet, G.D. (2004) Recommending STI vaccination to parents of adolescents, *Sexually Transmitted Diseases*, 31, 428–32.

Medical News Today (2007) Majority of US parents not in favor of HPV vaccine mandates. 27 May. http://www.medicalnewstoday.com/medicalnews.php?newsid=72302

Nathanson, C.A. (1991) *Dangerous Passage: the Social Control of Sexuality in Women's Adolescence.* Philadelphia: Temple University Press.

Nathanson, C.A. (2007) *Disease Prevention as Social Change.* New York: Russell Sage Foundation.

Nazeer, S. (2006) Screening for cervical cancer in developing countries. In Jordan, J.A. and Singer, A. (eds) *The Cervix.* 2nd edition. Blackwell Publishing.

NCSL (National Conference of State Legislatures) (2007) *HPV Vaccine.* See ncsl.org, 13 June.

Olshen, E., Woods, E.R., Austin, S.B. *et al.* (2005) Parental acceptance of the human papillomavirus vaccine, *Journal of Adolescent Health*, 37, 248–51.

Petryna, A., Lakoff, A. and Kleinman, A. (2006) *Global Pharmaceuticals: Ethics, Markets, Practices.* Durham, N.C.: Duke University Press.

Pollitt, K. (2005) Virginity or death! *The Nation*, 12 May.

Raley, J.C., Followwill, K.A., Zimet, G.D. and Ault, K.A. (2004) Gynecologists' attitudes regarding human papillomavirus vaccination: a survey of Fellows of the American College of Obstetricians and Gynecologists, *Infectious Diseases in Obstetrics and Gynecology*, 12, 3/4, 127–44.

Richert, C. (2005) Another medical culture war: how right-wing politics could keep a cancer vaccine off the market. CampusProgress.org, 13 December.

Risman, B. and Schwartz, P. (2002) After the sexual revolution: gender politics in teen dating, *Contexts*, 1, 1, 16–24.

Rubin, L. (1990) *Erotic Wars: What Happened to the Sexual Revolution?* New York: Farrar, Strauss and Giroux.

Sawaya, G.F. and Smith-McCune, K. (2007) HPV vaccination – more answers, more questions, *New England Journal of Medicine*, 356, 1991.

Schwarz, T.F. and Dubin, G.O. (2006) *An AS04-containing Human Papillomavirus (HPV) 16/18 Vaccine for Prevention of Cervical Cancer is Immunogenic and Well-tolerated in Women 15–55 Years Old.* Paper presented at the American Society of Clinical Oncology, Atlanta, GA.

Seidman, S. (1991) *Romantic Longings: Love in America, 1830–1980.* New York: Routledge.

Singer, A. and Jordan, J.A. (2006) The functional anatomy of the cervix, the cervical epithelium and the stroma. In Jordan, J.A. and Singer, A. (eds) The Cervix. 2nd edition. Malden: Blackwell Publishing.

Singer, A., Reid, B.L. and Coppleson, M. (1976) A hypothesis: the role of a high-risk male in the etiology of cervical carcinoma: a correlation of epidemiology and molecular biology, *American Journal of Obstetrics*, 126, 110–15.

Singh, G.K., Miller, B.A., Hankey, B.F. and Edwards, B.K. (2004) Persistent area socioeconomic disparities in US incidence of cervical cancer, mortality, stage, and survival, 1975–2000, *Cancer*, 101, 5, 1051–7.

Society for Adolescent Medicine (n.d.) Human papillomavirus (HPV) vaccine: a position statement of the Society for Adolescent Medicine. See www.adolescenthealth.org/PositionStatements.htm.

Stein, R. (2005) Cervical cancer vaccine gets injected with a social issue, *Washington Post*, 31 October.

Upchurch, D.M., Levy-Storms, L., Sucoff, C.A. and Aneshensel, C.S. (1998) Gender and ethnic differences in the timing of first sexual intercourse, *Family Planning Perspectives*, 30, 3, 121–7.

Van der Geest, S., Whyte, S.R. and Hardon, A. (1996) The anthropology of pharmaceuticals: a biographical approach, *Annual Review of Anthropology*, 25, 153–78.

Wardell, J. (2007) FDA denies Glaxo's cancer vaccine fast track status. *Associated Press*, 31 May.

Wheeler, C.M. (2007) Advances in primary and secondary interventions for cervical cancer: prophylactic human papillomavirus vaccines and testing, *Nature Clinical Practice Oncology*, 4, 4, 224–35.

Widmer, E., Treas, J. and Newcomb, R. (1998) Attitudes toward nonmarital sex in 24 countries, *Journal of Sex Research*, 34, 4, 349–58.

WHO (World Health Organization) (2006) Controversial new vaccine to prevent cervical cancer, www.who.int/bulletin/volumes/84/2/news20206/en/print.html.

Zimet, G.D. (2005) Improving adolescent health: focus on HPV vaccine acceptance, *Journal of Adolescent Health*, 37, S17–S23.

7

New forms of citizenship and socio-political inclusion: accessing antiretroviral therapy in a Rio de Janeiro *favela*

Fabian Cataldo

Introduction

Brazil was the first 'developing' or 'middle-income' country to implement free and universal distribution of antiretroviral therapy (ART), which successfully resulted in lowering AIDS morbidity and mortality rates throughout the country, and particularly in large urban centres (Ministério da Saúde 2004). In the early 1990s the World Bank predicted that by 2000, 1.2 million of Brazil's 186 million people would be infected with HIV; surveillance data suggest that 'only' about 600,000 Brazilians are infected (Okie 2006). Four main trends characterise the profile of the HIV epidemic in Brazil: the increase of infection in women, the increase of heterosexual transmission, the spread of the epidemic to regions outside large cities, and the increase in poor population groups (Galvão 2002, Ministério da Saúde 2008). Available epidemiological data on AIDS in Brazil show a clear breaking point in the evolution of the epidemic: 1996–1997 is a watershed period, before which there was a constant growth in the cumulative number of reported AIDS cases, and after which there is a distinctive decline (Ministério da Saúde 2003). These turning-point years correspond to the time when Brazil began to distribute ART on a 'universal' basis, free of charge at the point of access through its national health system, which continues to be one of the best-known parts of the Brazilian National AIDS Programme (NAP). The persistent negotiations between the Brazilian Ministry of Health and the pharmaceutical industry, together with the increase of the local production of generic drugs, contributed to a dramatic reduction in the price of antiretrovirals since 1996 (Okie 2006). These measures have been the focus of important press coverage and, in stark contrast with the South African example (Fassin 2006, Robins 2005), the Brazilian government is commonly portrayed as a 'pioneer' and 'leader' in the fight against HIV in low- and middle-income countries (Biehl 2006). The Brazilian NAP is now considered a model for other countries that need to put in place effective infrastructures to produce locally and provide access to antiretroviral drugs.

Given the international significance of the Brazilian approach, it is crucial to explore its effectiveness through a range of perspectives, and not simply through the national statistics currently available on overall mortality, morbidity and sexual behaviour. Whilst the ethical stance of the Brazilian programme has been widely applauded, there is a lack of empirical data on how the commitment to equitable and universal HIV prevention and treatment works in practice among the poorest population groups. Through an anthropological and observational research design, I proposed to explore the public health rhetoric of universalism, and assess the Brazilian programme primarily from the perspective of life in a *favela*[1] (shanty town) in Rio de Janeiro.

Drawing on Rabinow's concept of 'biosociality', defined as the forging of a collective identity under the emergent categories of biomedicine and allied sciences (Rabinow 1992, 1996), I refer to the idea of 'biosocial changes' to describe modifications in the life of an individual that relate to the interaction of biological and social forces, as illustrated in the work of Petryna (2002) and Nguyen (2005). I examine shifts in individual notions of social participation, and discuss how the 'medicalised body-self' may be linked to new citizenship claims for individuals treated for HIV and AIDS in the *favelas*.

I also refer to other new types of 'biopolitics' such as 'biological citizenship' (Petryna 2002, 2006, Rose and Novas 2005), and 'therapeutic citizenship' defined by Nguyen (2005, 2007) and Biehl (2004, 2006, 2007). In the wake of the Chernobyl disaster in post-Soviet Ukraine, Petryna (2002) examined the moral and political consequences of remedies available to locals and sufferers. Petryna tracked the emergence of what she calls a 'biological citizenship' through which sufferers stake claims for biomedical resources, social equity, and human rights. She defines 'biological citizenship' as both a collective and an individual survival strategy: a complex intersection of social institutions and the intense vulnerabilities of populations exposed to the determinations of the international political economy, also part of a larger story of democratisation and new structures of governance in post-socialist states (2002: 219). Rose and Novas (2005) also attest to the emergence of 'biological citizenship'. In common with Petryna, Rose and Novas characterise 'biological citizenship' as individualising to the extent that people shape their relations with themselves in terms of knowledge of their somatic individuality, and collectivising through biosocial groupings – a collectivism formed around a biological concept of shared identity (2005: 443). Nguyen (2005, 2007) and Biehl (2005, 2007) have also produced meaningful illustrations of the concept of 'biological citizenship' and have used the idea of 'therapeutic citizenship' to describe the way in which people living with HIV (PLHIV) appropriate ART as a set of rights and responsibilities to negotiate these at times of conflicting moral economies (Nguyen 2007), resulting in a system of claims and ethical projects that arise out of the conjugation of techniques used to govern populations and manage individual bodies (Nguyen 2005).

My intention in this chapter is to illustrate how emerging claims to citizenship and bio-political inclusion are associated with accessing ART in a low-income population group, and how they may be understood as a series of claims made on a global social order on the basis of a therapeutic predicament (Nguyen 2005). I describe how a series of biosocial changes are formed and articulated within a specific socio-political setting and in relation to prevailing forms of structural violence. Bio-political debates were largely developed in European and North American contexts, or in relation to observations made within NGOs and institutional settings. I aim to show how these notions might be equally relevant in a low-income 'marginalised' population in a non-Western and non-institutional setting, namely in the context of accessing HIV treatment in Brazil's *favelas*.

Methods

The methodology used needs to be contextualised within the specific nature of fieldwork in the *favelas* of Rio de Janeiro; observations were limited by the perilous conditions of the chosen location, and by the sensitive nature of topics such as HIV and related therapeutic issues. The research is based on 13 months of anthropological fieldwork in Brazil. The bulk of the fieldwork took place in a *favela* close to the *Centro* of Rio de Janeiro, in the neighbourhood of Santa Teresa. This *favela* was selected because of its relative accessibility, although violence and the presence of armed gangs were great impediments to the progress and completion of fieldwork. An estimated 10,000 individuals live in this *favela*. Through participant observation of daily life and informal conversation with inhabitants, it was possible to place issues around health, treatment and equity, in local context. Over a period of five months, I followed a team at the local health centre *(Centro Municipal de Saúde)* composed of paediatricians, psychologists, counsellors, and social workers, as they organised a series of activities on health and disease prevention for teenagers living in the *favela*.

Additional observation in NGOs was conducted through participation in the activities of two local organisations working in the field of HIV, whose work is directly linked to low-income population groups in Rio: CEDAPS (Centre for Health Promotion) and Grupo Pela Vidda Rio (GPV – Group for the value, integration, and dignity of people living with AIDS). Three focus groups were conducted at CEDAPS with a group of 15 women living in different *favelas* in Rio. These meetings were organised with the aim of collecting a range of spontaneous definitions of structural problems, and to provide data on a wide spectrum of experiences related to health, illness, health care, and HIV in other *favelas* throughout the city. Over a period of seven months with CEDAPS, I worked closely with a group of women who ran the *Núcleos Comunitários de Prevenção das DST/AIDS* (STD/AIDS Community Prevention Centres) and local health-promotion teams in 15 different *favelas* of Rio. I also participated in the activities of Grupo Pela Vidda (GPV) where I regularly took part in meetings for a support group of around 30 participants living with HIV.

A number of research participants were identified throughout that period and later interviewed. Snowball and opportunistic sampling methods were used to identify 25 research participants. Their life histories, narratives of illness, and in-depth semi-structured interviews were collected during the second phase of the fieldwork. In addition, key informant interviews were conducted with 16 NGO workers and 12 health practitioners from local health centres and hospitals. The interviews addressed different issues according to the research participants' circumstances, but each was broadly organised around a set of topics referring to experience of HIV therapies, health and illness, socio-economic situation, family and household composition, education and local politics. It was not possible, for the purpose of this chapter, to provide as many facts and details about each of the informants and their specific circumstances as I would have wished. Instead, I have deliberately selected a number of topics from my fieldwork observation, and retained only those issues directly connected to my overall argument. Individual names and locations have been modified in this script to comply with the relevant ethical guidelines[2] on confidentiality and protection of informants against potential harm as a consequence of the research.

Political alienation and renewed marginalisation

The experiences of accessing ART that I describe through my observation within the *favelas* of Rio de Janeiro are only intelligible in the light of experiences of stigmatisation and structural violence. One of the key social problems in Rio de Janeiro is the lack of progress in improving the distribution of income. Regional income inequalities have pushed thousands of migrants from rural to urban areas over the last few decades throughout Brazil, which led to the expansion and development of new *favelas*, mainly in large cities. In Rio de Janeiro, wealth disparities are particularly prominent and the city is composed of a patchwork of poor and wealthy neighbourhoods living side by side. Today, there are more than 750 *favelas* in Rio de Janeiro, with approximately 1.65 million inhabitants (Perlman 2005).

Although significant variations in income levels exist both within the *favelas* and in other neighbourhoods, the great majority of *favela* residents have few financial resources and live in poor housing conditions. The *favelas* have changed over the past 100 years; most houses are now made of bricks, connected to electricity since the end of the 1970s, and have had water as well as sewerage systems since the 1980s (Zaluar and Alvito 2003). Whilst the *favelas* have gradually increased the quality of their urban amenities and expanded in size, progress is slow, however, and today's *favelas* face a novel set of difficulties, such as the recurring conflicts resulting from the presence of the drug traffic. Throughout most of the 20th century, the *favelas* were singled out as places propitious to the development of disease and bad hygiene (Valladares 2005). More recently, numerous *favelas* have become 'extra-territorial zones' controlled by drug traffickers, where the absence of public authorities (federal, state, or municipal) is almost complete (Inciardi *et al.* 2000). To that extent, the 'narcotization' (the increase of the influence of narcotic drugs) of Rio's *favelas*, in conjunction with the militarisation of the drug traffic since the progressive introduction of cocaine over the last 25 years (Dowdney 2003), has significantly reinforced the isolation of these neighbourhoods, now commonly labelled as dangerous and unsafe. The presence of the drug trafficking has not only renewed, but also intensified, a process of marginalisation of the *favelas* and their inhabitants. The simple fact of living in a *favela*, say many of the local inhabitants, is enough to be seen as a marginal. A *favelado*, literally 'the inhabitant of a *favela'*, has become a pejorative term, which some *favela* inhabitants themselves find offensive, as it is commonly linked to negative perceptions of the *favelas*. Nevertheless, through employment, education, consumption, social life and leisure activities, *favela* residents are far from confined to the territory of their own neighbourhood, and are fully involved in the daily life of the rest of the city (Perlman 1976, Zaluar 2002, Valladares 2005). This constant flow of people between the interior and exterior of the *favelas* constitutes one of the most striking aspects of the social, political, cultural, and economic life of Rio de Janeiro.

In the *favela* Morro dos Reis, on the hillsides of Santa Teresa in Rio, local people often express feelings of impotence towards the ubiquitous violence that they experience. The ongoing struggle for control between the police and drug traffickers has profound consequences for both local inhabitants and for the organisation of the *favela* in general. Locals perceive the control held by drug factions over their neighbourhood to be in conflict with their individual civil rights. On the other side of the 'battlefield', as they label their own neighbourhood, the frequent and brusque invasions by police forces such as the *BOPE*[3] leave inhabitants stressed, traumatised, and feeling vulnerable (Dowdney 2003). Unable to rely on either side, the same individuals feel largely ignored and 'abandoned' by the local authorities and by their government for their lack of intervention in improving the situation. Harris (1994) shows how, in a different Latin-American setting, violence is explicitly treated as a necessary alternative state rather than a breakdown of normality. In the Brazilian context, seemingly, violence is a 'plural subject' (Kleinman 2000). Its definition varies according to various situational circumstances but also, and perhaps more importantly, in relation to a watershed between *favelas* and middle class experiences. Widespread definitions of violence among *Cariocas* (inhabitants of Rio de Janeiro) encompass criminal behaviour, the use of physical force, aggression, domestic violence, and the actions of drug traffic (Penglase 2005). *Favela* inhabitants, in addition to the latter, very often use the term 'violence' as a substitute for 'the drug trade' at large. Feldman (1991) described how the body is used, commodified and injured to serve nationalist discourse in the process of civil war in Northern Ireland. In the same way, the violence resulting from the presence of the drug trade within *favela* neighbourhoods induces a particular form of political violence. This violence is constantly re-enacted through the concatenation of forced dependency on the traffic, menace and threat, and it is also inflicted by the drug commandos' ubiquitous presence as they constantly watch and control the *favela's* entrances.

This political form of violence and the feelings of impotence that it creates among locals have taken root quickly in the *favelas* because the state (national and regional) has been unsuccessful in asserting and sustaining its authority, both in political and economic terms, among these neighbourhoods. Penglase (2005) shows how local drug gangs have repeatedly used tactics such as the 'shutdown of Rio de Janeiro' as a way of demonstrating that the city's drug traffickers possess a power that the local authorities do not have: new forms of power are being constructed, and a new type of war conducted, at the very moment when there is a deep, region-wide disenchantment with democracy, and when the role of the state as the central economic and political actor is increasingly being called into question (Penglase 2005). Thus, today *favela* inhabitants find themselves involved in a political form of marginalisation which, unlike any previous forms of marginality (Perlman 1976), is deeply embedded in a political form of violence that results from the absence of sustained intervention from the state to tackle the growth of the drug trade.

Taking ART in the favelas

The specificities of the local context described above proved to be central to *favela* inhabitants' experience of taking ART. The *favela* Morro dos Reis has been Valedio's family home for the last 20 years. Now aged 48, he was born near Recife, in one of Brazil's North East poorest neighbourhoods. After his parents' separation when he was 12, his mother moved to Rio de Janeiro to find a job. Valedio moved to Rio a few months later with his three brothers and sisters. There he had to give up school, and worked in a succession of manual jobs, first as a cleaner and then in retail. At 12, he already felt like a grown man, he says, as he needed to work for himself and 'fight for his own life'. When he was 13 he met his future wife, a young woman also from the North East called Paula. She is a couple of years older than he is, and they had their first child a year after they met. Valedio's life changed dramatically at 18 when he was convicted for robbery and was sent to jail for nine years. In 2002, he discovered after an operation to remove a cyst that he was infected with HIV and hepatitis C. His wife Paula tested HIV positive a few weeks after he received his diagnosis. Both of them have been taking antiretrovirals for four years. They are followed-up regularly – once every three months – by the lung specialist at the local health centre, from where they also collect their antiretroviral drugs and test results.

Similarly to other research participants on ART, although Valedio and Paula said they took ART as prescribed by their physician, it became apparent with time that they did not adhere, either occasionally or regularly, to their treatment. The most frequent reason given for the temporary cessation of treatment seems to be the recurrence of various side effects. In some cases, because side effects can affect one's capacity to go to work, the treatment itself is seen as the source of illness, and non-adherence to the therapy was seen as one of few options available when work is a means of survival in the short term; for many PLHIV in the *favelas*, adhering to ART is a 'luxury' that poor people simply cannot afford because however strongly the side effects may affect their body, they need to carry on and work to make a living. In-depth interviews and participant observation showed that *favela* inhabitants involved in the research, regardless of their age, gender, family, and racial background, see a strong connection between the concept of 'illness' and that of 'immobility' or 'paralysis' of the body. An individual suffering from an illness is broadly defined as someone whose physical ability to move or walk is seriously impaired. Importantly, given that illness is seen as an impairment affecting mobility, it is also identified in connection with one's ability to work, or more precisely to go to work. In the Morro dos Reis *favela*, because local definitions of illness are closely linked to work and mobility, they also become a significant factor in the success of treatment for HIV. The asymptomatic nature of HIV infection and its relatively slow development in the body means that, in the context of the *favelas*, any illness or complications related to HIV are generally not taken care of, unless they interfere with a PLHIV's mobility and daily activities.

Another reason PLHIV gave for missing some of the daily doses of treatment is related to alcohol consumption. They say some of the pills are not compatible with beer, and explained to me why they deliberately omit to take them during weekends, since this is the time of the week when they tend to drink more alcohol. Respondents also often described the treatment they are receiving, the appearance of the drugs and their functions in a number of ways. These descriptions were associated with the physical attributes of the drugs, such as their colour, shape, and boxes, and often pills were associated with a physiological need and were linked to the time of the day when they were taken. Some of the drugs that must be taken in the evening were described as helping them sleep, while the daytime pills helped one to feel hungry or maintain a certain level of physical activity.

An important observation is that even when research participants missed doses of ART, some on a regular basis, they continued to pick up the drugs from the local health centre at regular intervals, as required by their prescription, but either kept the extra pills at home, or gave away the surplus to one of the local Evangelical churches. A few of those I met had also started to share or exchange antiretroviral drugs between themselves. Valedio and Paula, for instance, said that they were being given too much medicine to treat themselves and their bodies could not possibly cope with such a large quantity of drugs. At some point, Paula decided to stop collecting her own treatment from the local health centre and she started to use her husband's drugs to 'help him get through them'.

A local definition of 'illness' strongly linked to the ability to work is not exclusive to *favela* neighbourhoods but has serious consequences in the context of HIV treatment. One of the immediate consequences of illness being so closely defined by the capacity/incapacity to work, is that *favela* residents tend to seek medical advice in the later stages of 'disease' development. Herbal and home remedies are preferred until worrying symptoms appear; that is when mobility is significantly affected, or when one is unable to go to work. Seeking medical help at the later stages of disease development, as well as late diagnosis, has some consequences on HIV prevalence and increases the risks of individuals unaware of their seropositivity infecting others through unprotected sex. In terms of mortality, late diagnoses as a consequence of symptomatic manifestations of AIDS and opportunistic illnesses, means that HIV has already significantly weakened the immune system. Lower rates for HIV testing which were reported within *favelas* (Ministério da Saúde 2002) might be explained by this phenomenon, at least partially.

New biosocialities

Elza is a good-looking, tall, 22-year-old woman, who lives in the *favela* with her six-year-old son, Pedro. Four years ago, she was diagnosed HIV positive when she was treated for meningitis. Elza does not want the rest of her neighbourhood to know about her serostatus, and she is frightened that she could face discrimination or rejection if it becomes known she is HIV positive. She said that, within her *favela*, access to health care is extremely poor. In contrast, she thinks that the level of health care she receives for HIV is very good, as for other poor people. She considers the service that deals with HIV to be better organised, more efficient, and more reliable than the rest of the public health-care system. She stressed that she was lucky to be living in Brazil because they have the NAP. Importantly, her experience of being treated and receiving antiretrovirals via a public health policy seems to be linked to positive opinions about the government: 'I think the government is good, very good, it continues to make medicine available for us, I think it has to continue to do so'.

Originally from Fortaleza, Edilson arrived in Rio aged 16, in search of work and 'better days' as he put it. Now aged 47, he still lives in one of the *favelas* and works for eight to nine hours a day selling drinks and refreshments on the beach. He recently joined an HIV support group shortly after testing HIV positive a few months earlier. As did everyone else I interviewed or met who was on ART, Edilson often brought up issues about the price of antiretrovirals, insisting that the drugs he received were extremely costly, and that he would not be able to afford the drugs if he had to pay for them. Like many others, he often compared his situation with that of people in other Latin American countries where there was no similar public health policy for AIDS, and said he felt 'privileged' to be living in Brazil.

It was observed during fieldwork that taking antiretrovirals and being involved in the NAP via local health centres and NGO interventions might encourage new forms of bio-sociality for PLHIV in the *favelas*. In spite of the fact that many *favela* inhabitants feel discriminated against for being poor, less educated, for hailing from other regions, and for being stigmatised by the ongoing violence resulting from the growing narco-trafficking, being treated through the NAP seemed to provide a relative experience of 'inclusion' into the larger socio-political order. All the informants on ART were aware that they received their antiretrovirals through a public health policy managed by the national government, and they were also aware that Brazil's neighbouring countries did not provide free ART to their citizens (as of 2005). PLHIV recognise that the Brazilian Ministry of Health has put in place a complex logistical effort to give people access to treatment through the existing National Health System (SUS), and that it has developed a nationwide strategy to distribute antiretroviral drugs and monitor ART. Also, it became clear through fieldwork observations that the government's efforts to produce locally some of the generics used in the composition of ART over the last 10 years were widely acknowledged by PLHIV. Research participants living with HIV and taking antiretrovirals, talked repeatedly about their pride in seeing their own government defy the pharmaceutical 'giants' in order to lower the cost of existing treatments and to sustain the availability of antiretroviral drugs.

It was also observed during this study that access to ART for some *favela* inhabitants living with HIV has influenced individual perceptions about, and personal relations to, the medical system as a whole. PLHIV attend their health centre regularly, once every other month on average, and through regular visits to a local health centre, individuals on ART have developed close relationships with health practitioners (nurses, doctors, pharmacist, social workers, administrative staff). Some also told me that since they had started ART, they had become more disposed to use biomedical drugs as a first recourse instead of using home-made remedies. These individuals said that they had started to consult a doctor more spontaneously, without allowing the early symptoms, however benign, to worsen to the point of being perceived as 'worrying symptoms' or being 'immobilised'.

Similarly, PLHIV in the *favelas* have developed better skills in identifying where to get further assistance, for instance through the contact they have with local NGOs working in the field of HIV. People on ART appeared to be more disposed to seek help and support from one of the NGOs specialising in HIV. Not only do these groups provide participants with new social networks formed of other participants and NGO staff members, but they also represent the synapses of the AIDS political activism throughout the country. These are places where people can find support and through which many of them become more sensitive to their individual rights. My observations suggest that through these various meetings, workshops, courses, and local support groups, PLHIV involved in these environments are exhorted both implicitly and explicitly to claim further rights to receive treatment, to obtain financial compensation, to be involved in decision-making processes, to achieve greater social inclusion, to reduce stigma in the workplace and within families, to gain further rights (such as access to free public transport) and, importantly, to do so on the basis of their therapeutic needs.

Politicised bodies

As described earlier, a large portion of *favela* residents expressed experiences of 'exclusion', felt 'excluded' from public policies and had lost faith in politicians, who had 'let them down' along with the rest of the population on many issues, including social exclusion, violence and unemployment. By focusing on *favela* residents living with HIV and taking ART, I suggest that the NAP has contributed to lessening the existing pervasive negative attitudes towards the national state[4] and its representatives. In-depth interviews and case studies indicate that *favela* inhabitants taking ART seem to adopt more sympathetic views towards their government and its representatives, as they endorse the work of the Ministry of Health and express sympathy for the politicians who were involved in the implementation of the NAP.

ART works as a constant reminder of how much one's survival relies on the availability of the drugs and, consequently, on the sustainability of the very public health programme that provides the population with free access to them. Research participants expressed their fears that their government would not be able to sustain its policy of free and widespread distribution of ART. 'I am afraid that we could be in a situation where treatment is not available any more, and if there is a lack of treatment it would be fatal, death would be the only outcome [. . .] I'm scared, because I have seen many weaknesses in the government, and I'm scared that it could be another failure' said Edilson during an interview. Each of the research participants living with HIV and taking antiretrovirals expressed the feeling of dependence on the government because of their medical treatment. On the one hand, they feel grateful that they can access free-of-charge treatment through the public system and, on the other, they are afraid of having to pay for treatment in the future. They often said that their individual health and perspectives about the future depended on the performance of the country. Importantly, they also felt that they were more vulnerable than other individuals with HIV who did not live in *favela*s, because if ART stopped being available for free, they could not afford to pay for it, nor could they move to another country to receive treatment.

Thus, in the local context of *favela* neighbourhoods, receiving antiretrovirals via the public health system is translated by *favela* residents themselves into a right to receive treatment like any other citizen, regardless of wealth distribution and socio-economic disparities, but it is also understood as a relation of dependency on a state programme, namely the NAP, and on the stability of the political system as a whole. Among PLHIV living in the *favelas*, a relationship of reliance is established between the 'sick' body and the state, and the chances of staying alive are envisaged in relation to the degree of sustainability of the NAP itself. In that sense, antiretroviral drugs are perceived as a direct 'link' between the individual body and the state. Because of the strong side effects, *favela* residents consider that antiretrovirals affect and, in some cases, incapacitate their ability to work and live normally. Hence, the drugs also evoke feelings of suspicion about their 'invasive' nature, and they are seen as intrusive and alien to people's lives, because they are often accompanied by important changes in the social and professional lives of those receiving the treatment.

In addition, through the treatment they receive and related services which they have access to (support groups, counselling, legal advice, housing services, workshops), the same *favela* inhabitants become exposed and sometimes affiliated to new social environments (Galvão 2000). For instance, in Morro dos Reis, those who are unable to pick up their treatment from the health centre receive them via a postal service organised by the National Health System (SUS). Carla, a local volunteer, ensures that every parcel is delivered as she regularly goes around the neighbourhood to 'check in' on those receiving treatment. The interactions between Carla and other *favela* inhabitants is one of the examples which illustrates how distribution of treatment and the work of local volunteers trained by a local NGO (CEDAPS) creates therapeutic networks within the *favela*, or between the health-care system and *favela* inhabitants. Hence, the 'social body' of *favela* residents on ART is also deeply affected by the AIDS policy, and numerous new social networks are progressively formed from the association of people infected and affected by HIV. Local NGOs play a central role in the formation of these new networks, which they continue to influence through their work as political activists and through their role as the leaders of the so-called 'social control' in the field of HIV.[5] Since the early 1980s, NGOs have radically influenced Brazil's response to HIV; today they work together with the NAP in a dynamic characterised by great tensions – protests and unrest – and collaboration (for instance to distribute condoms and prevention leaflets among men who have sex with men, transvestites and transsexuals, sex workers, and in the *favelas*).

In Latin America, 'access to citizenship' is often turned into a synonym for 'access to an ideal world', and promoted as such by social militants, including NGOs, international and governmental organisations (Sorj 2004). In the absence of durable positive intervention by the state in the *favelas*, egalitarian movements such as those first described by Marshall (1950, 1964) materialise on the ground through the work of NGOs. Although local NGO projects do not generally aim to be universal, have specific goals, and rely on particular methods and ideologies, they also constitute, for inhabitants in the Morro dos Reis *favela* and others, one of the only palpable and positive interventions to alleviate problems affecting the local population such as the lack of education, illiteracy, lack of professional skills, unemployment, lack of health care, lack of food, discrimination, and lack of political participation. In the 'absence' of sustained state interventions in the *favelas*, NGOs have become powerful political actors and manage to provide a few *favela* inhabitants with some of the basic services that the state has failed to deliver. The activities of local NGOs such as CEDAPS and GPV, who both support PLHIV at the local level, illustrate the extent to which PLHIV gain greater awareness of political activism in the domain of HIV treatment and health care. Through regular workshops, support groups, visits to households, and numerous meetings, trainings, or buddy-type programmes, both GPV and CEDAPS contribute actively in informing and influencing local opinions about rights activism, by encouraging its participants to interrogate ideas around access to treatment, citizenship, and human rights.

Conclusions

The singularity of the therapeutic options offered to *favela* inhabitants taking ART, and thus the singularity of their 'therapeutic economy' (Nguyen 2005), is defined on the one hand by the availability of free treatment and medical assistance through the Brazilian public health system and, on the other, by access to a range of social services and discourses about citizenship through new social networks linked to accessing ART and local AIDS activism. I illustrated how, in the context of Rio's *favelas*, PLHIV's perspectives on socio-political inclusion are influenced by their involvement in this new therapeutic economy, and how a number of PLHIV's claims to greater socio-political participation is profoundly intertwined with their novel access to HIV treatment and care. I have argued that accessing ART and other HIV-related services, via the public health system and local NGOs, results in biosocial changes and greater involvement in new or existing therapeutic environments, which allow individuals to enjoy the right (with an emphasis on 'having rights') to therapies and treatments. This 'right to health' and right to accessing ART must be understood within the perspective of the formation of the Brazilian National Health System (SUS) in the 1980s, in which the concept of 'health' itself is defined as a basic human right and a basis for citizenship.

The distinctiveness of the local biosocial changes generated by the Brazilian NAP resides in the inclusive attribute of the programme which facilitates access to expensive antiretroviral drugs through the National Health System, whilst access to virtually any other types of public intervention seems to be increasingly difficult and sometimes impossible from the perspective of *favela* inhabitants. Similarly to Farmer's (1992) findings regarding 'conspiracy theories' in Haiti, local reactions to the NAP – and not only to the local health services – reveal sophisticated readings of the 'nation-state' and international efforts at health intervention. These include contradictory understandings, which endorse the timely and accessible health interventions set up by the government, but which simultaneously involve feelings of suspicion towards an alien, interfering state, practising discrimination against a poor and expendable population. Hence, the NAP actually exceeds the design of the public health programme itself, as people also rely very much on the existence of a 'moral economy', along the lines of Farmer's (2003) definition of health as a basic human right, and claim further rights on the basis of their medicalised body-self.

The notion of 'therapeutic citizenship' allows us to conceptualise the medicalised body as a platform for the formation and development of new claims about the right to health jointly with new attitudes towards socio-political inclusion and citizenship. 'Therapeutic citizenship' is however only meaningful when considered through a close examination of the complexities of grounded social interactions. As I have illustrated, notions of social participation and citizenship are embedded in a deep and complex history of exclusion towards *favela* residents, and the therapeutic economy of PLHIV living in the *favelas* must be understood within this context. The unique nature of therapeutic citizenship in the *favelas* resides in the history of the struggle to achieve greater inclusion into the rest of society throughout the 20th century, to improve their living conditions and to alleviate some of the structural violence that affects their daily lives. In the context of this specific political economy, and unlike previous forms of socio-political mobilisation attempted by *favela* inhabitants, 'therapeutic citizenship' translates into a more focused, more conspicuous, and more tangible set of claims and concerns organised around the individual body-self and related to the right to health, the availability of free drugs and treatment, and the sustainability of public health policies.

Notes

1   The term 'favela' is used in Brazil to designate 'shanty towns'. Many local inhabitants would favour the appellation 'comunidade' (community) over the term 'favela' to refer to their own neighbourhood, whilst others choose to use the appellation 'favela' as a means of affirmation of a distinct identity.

2   Association of Social Anthropologists of the UK and the Commonwealth (1999 [1987]), World Medical Association Declaration of Helsinki (2002 [1964]), and The Wellcome Trust (Alderson 2001).

3   *Batalhão de Operações Especias*, a special branch of the police force trained to deal with armed conflicts and drug factions.
4   Defined here as the body politic constituting a nation.
5   In this context, the use of the term 'social control' *(controle social)* refers to a common use of the term in Brazil as the process through which 'civil society' (in its broadest sense) can, and must, exercise a constant and critical examination of the decisions and actions emanating from the executive, legislative and judicial powers, or from other governmental bodies and their representatives.

References

Alderson, P. (2001) *On doing Qualitative Research linked to Healthcare.* 2 vols. London: The Wellcome Trust.

Association of Social Anthropologists of the UK and the Commonwealth (1999 [1987]) *Ethical Guidelines for Good Research Practice.* London.

Biehl, J. (2004) The activist state. Global pharmaceuticals, AIDS, and citizenship in Brazil, *Social Text*, 22, 3, 105–32.

Biehl, J. (2005) Technologies of Invisibility: Politics of Life and Social Inequality. In Inda, J.X. (ed.) *Anthropologies of Modernity: Foucault, Governmentality, and Life Politics.* Oxford: Blackwell Publishing.

Biehl, J. (2006) Pharmaceutical governance. In Petryna, A., Lakoff, A. and Kleinman, A. (eds) *Global Pharmaceuticals. Ethics, Markets, Practices.* Durham and London: Duke University Press.

Biehl, J. (2007) *Will to Live: AIDS Therapies and the Politics of Survival.* Princeton: Princeton University Press.

Dowdney, L. (2003) *Children of the Drug Trade. A Case Study of Children in Organised Armed Violence in Rio de Janeiro.* Rio de Janeiro: Viveiros de Castro Editora.

Farmer, P. (1992) *AIDS and Accusation; Haiti and the Geography of Blame.* Berkeley: University of California Press.

Farmer, P. (2003) *Pathologies of Power. Health, Human Rights, and the New War on the Poor.* Berkeley: University of California Press.

Fassin, D. (2006) *Quand les corps se souviennent. Expériences et politiques du SIDA en Afrique du Sud.* Paris: La Découverte.

Feldman, A. (1991) *Formations of Violence: the Narrative of the Body and Political Terror in Northern Ireland.* Chicago: University of Chicago Press.

Galvão, J. (2002) Access to Antiretroviral Drugs in Brazil, *The Lancet*, 360, 9348, 1862–5.

Harris, O. (1994) Condor and bull: the ambiguities of masculinity in Northern Potosí. In Harvey, P. and Gow, P. (eds) *Sex and Violence.* London: Routledge.

Inciardi, J., Surratt, H. and Telles, P. (2000) *Sex, Drugs, and HIV/AIDS in Brazil.* Boulder, CO: Westview Press.

Kleinman, A. (2000) The violences of everyday life: the multiple forms and dynamics of social violence. In Das, V., Kleinman, A., Ramphele, M. and Reynolds, P. (eds) *Violence and Subjectivity.* Berkeley and Los Angeles: University of California Press.

Marshall, T.H. (1950) *Citizenship and Social Class, and Other Essays.* London: Cambridge University Press.

Marshal, T.H. (1964) *Class, Citizenship, and Social Development.* Chicago, London: The University of Chicago Press.

Ministério da Saúde (2002) Dados epidemiológicos – Brasil. *Boletim epidemiológico AIDS*, ANO XVI, 1, 17–34.

Ministério da Saúde (2003) *Boletim epidemiológico AIDS*, ANO XVII (01).

Ministério da Saúde (2004, 2008) *Resposta. A Experiência do Programa Brasileiro de Aids.* São Paulo: Governo Federal, Brasil.

Nguyen, V. (2005) Antiretroviral globalism, biopolitics, and therapeutic citizenship. In Ong, A. and Collier, S.J. (eds) *Global Assemblages: Technology, Politics, and Ethics as Anthropological Problems.* Oxford: Blackwell Publishing.

Nguyen, V. *et al.* (2007) *Adherence as Therapeutic Citizenship: Impact of the History of Access to Antiretroviral Drugs on Adherence to Treatment.* AIDS 21, Supplement 5, S31–S35.

Okie, S. (2006) Fighting HIV – Lessons from Brazil, *New England Journal of Medicine*, 349, 19, 1977–81.

Penglase, B. (2005) The Shutdown of Rio de Janeiro, *Anthropology Today*, 21, October, 3–6.

Perlman, J. (1976) *The Myth of Marginality. Urban Poverty and Politics in Rio de Janeiro.* Berkeley: University of California Press.

Perlman, J. (2005) The myth of marginality revisited. The case of *Favelas* in Rio de Janeiro, 1969–2003. In Hanley, L.M., Ruble, B.A. and Tulchin, J.S. (eds) *Becoming Global and the New Poverty of Cities.* Washington DC: Woodrow Wilson International Center for Scholars.

Petryna, A. (2002) *Life Exposed: Biological Citizens after Chernobyl.* Princeton: Princeton University Press.

Petryna, A. (2006) Globalizing human subjects research. In Petryna, A., Lakoff, A. and Kleinman, A. (eds) *Global Pharmaceuticals. Ethics, Markets, Practices.* Durham and London: Duke University Press.

Rabinow. P. (1992) Artificiality and enlightenment: from sociobiology to biosociality. In Crary, J. and Kwinter, S. (eds) *Incorporations.* New York: Zone.

Rabinow P. (1996) *Essays on the Anthropology of Reason.* Princeton NJ: Princeton University Press.

Robins, S. (2005) The politics of ambiguity in a time of AIDS, *Sunday Independent*, 6 March.

Rose, N. and Novas, C. (2005) Biological citizenship. In Ong, A. and Collier, S.J. (eds) *Global Assemblages: Technology, Politics, and Ethics as Anthropological Problems.* Oxford: Blackwell Publishing.

Sorj, B. (2004) *A Democracia Inesperada: Cidadania, Direitos Humans e Desigualdade Social.* Rio de Janeiro: Jorge Zahar.

Valladares, L. do Prado (2005) *A Invenção da Favela: do Mito de Origem a Favela.com.* Rio de Janeiro: FGV.

World Medical Association (2002 [1964]) *World Medical Association Declaration of Helsinki. Ethical Principles for Medical Research Involving Human Subjects.*

Zaluar, A. (2002 [1985]) *A Máquina e a Revolta; As Organizções Populares e o Significado da Pobreza.* São Paulo: Brasiliense.

Zaluar, A. and Alvito, M. (eds) (2003 [1998]) *Um Século de Favela.* Rio de Janeiro: Fundação Getulio Vargas.

8

Over-the-counter medicines: professional expertise and consumer discourses

Fiona A. Stevenson, Miranda Leontowitsch and Catherine Duggan

Introduction

Ideas of participation and partnership in health-care consultations have attracted increasing attention in recent years, particularly in England. The consequences in terms of the necessary shifts in existing relationships are, however, often overlooked. This chapter examines how pharmacists work to maintain their professional expertise against the rise of health-care consumerism where an increasingly informed customer is encouraged to engage in self-care and to participate in decisions about treatment.

We consider consultations in the UK between pharmacists and customers for over-the-counter (OTC) medicines. Potential conflicts between professional expertise and consumer discourses may be brought into sharp relief by OTC medicines. This is because OTC medicines may be perceived by customers to require expert advice or, alternatively, may be viewed as a commodity depending on the medicine involved and the particular context within which medicine is sought.

Initially, we examine the recent thinking concerned with public participation in health care and models of participation. This provides a context for then considering professional expertise and health-care consumerism within the pharmacy setting.

Participation in health care

The notion of partnership has been central to UK health policy for over 10 years (Milewa, Dowswell and Harrison 2002) and is a key element of the UK Labour Government's modernisation agenda (Newman and Vidler 2006). A plethora of policies evokes models of practice such as shared information, shared evaluation, shared decision making, and shared responsibilities (Department of Health (DoH) 1996, 1999, 2000a, 2001a, 2001b, 2001c, 2003a). The term 'concordance' was coined in the late 1990s to describe a model of practice with an emphasis on partnership and in particular the importance of taking account of lay views. The ultimate goal was to reduce non-adherence to medicines. Concordance was endorsed in the policy document *Pharmacy in the Future* (DoH 2000a).

Policy documentation in the UK (see DoH 2005) contains a clear expectation that pharmacists should work with customers to aid decisions about self-care and OTC medicines. Moreover, recommendations on encouraging public participation in health are supported by the ever increasing availability of sources of advice and information on minor illnesses and medication. Such information is available from health-care sites such as pharmacies. Other sources of information include the media, Internet and friends and family. Yet, research on encounters between doctors and patients suggests that availability of information does not necessarily mean patients identify themselves as 'informed patients'. Henwood *et al.* (2003) raised three constraints: (i) people may be reluctant to take on the responsibility implied by the 'informed patient' discourse; (ii) problems with health literacy; and (iii) there may be constraints in the medical encounter itself which further inhibit empowerment through information. Moreover, although patients possess expertise in relation to their own experiences, their views and beliefs may not be consistent with medical thinking. It is therefore important not to confuse the use and manipulation of technical knowledge (the realm of expertise) with the worthy political aim of ensuring participation and consultation of the lay public in matters to do with medicines (Prior 2003).

Having provided a brief overview of recent thinking in relation to participation in health care, it is important to consider the other side of the health-care relationship, namely professional expertise. This provides a context for considering roles in the relationship between pharmacists and customers.

Pharmacists' professional expertise

Concerns about the role and professional status of pharmacists have been voiced over a period of more than 40 years (*cf.* Denzin and Metlin 1966, Dingwall and Wilson 1995, Harding and Taylor 1997). For community pharmacists, concerns about role and professional status were brought into particular relief by the loss to industry of their technical role of compounding drugs. The role and professional status of community pharmacists was specifically tackled in the Nuffield Report (1986) with the suggestion of an extended role for community pharmacists, relating in particular to giving health advice. The idea of an extended role reappeared more recently in the new Community Pharmacy Contract and documents such as *Choosing Health through Pharmacy* (DoH 2005).

Harding and Taylor (1997), however, argued that medicines have to remain the centre of pharmacists' services if pharmacy is to remain a profession. This is because the fundamental nature of pharmaceutical expertise is control over the symbolic transformation of the pharmacological entity – the drug – into the social object – the medicine. Pharmacists have a publicly recognised authority to supply pharmacological entities which because they are provided by an 'expert' become imbued with meaning as medicines. They used the example of aspirin to demonstrate how the provision of advice and selection of a particular medicine by pharmacists may invest even medicines regarded as familiar with additional value and status. They argued that:

> (. . .) aspirin can be regarded as a commodity widely available to the public as a panacea for mild to moderate pain. In such circumstances aspirin is loaded with no more symbolic significance than any other product available from retail outlets such as supermarkets or petrol filling stations, because it is supplied beyond the surveillance of drug 'experts'. However, when aspirin is selected (from a range of alternative drugs) by an 'expert', sanctioned to interpret its appropriateness for a specific individual, this commonly available drug has the potential to be symbolically transformed into a medicine. This process may benefit the public by investing a product with added value, in that a specific drug is targeted to their specific requirements. Additionally, the process may benefit pharmacists by fostering a greater utilisation of, and dependence on, their drug knowledge by the public (Harding and Taylor 1997: 554).

This quotation highlights how the location of sale of a medicine has the potential to affect the way it is viewed by the consumer. The association between location of advice giving and professionalism is also apparent in the recent encouragement for pharmacists to have separate areas or a room for conducting consultations (DoH 2005).

The National Pharmaceutical Association (NPA), which represents community pharmacists, has argued that availability of medicines should be restricted on the basis that 'medicines are not consumer goods and should not be treated like any other commodity' (NPA 2007). In reality, however, there is an increasing availability of drugs for purchase from non-pharmacy outlets with the associated inference that no accompanying 'expert' supervision and advice is necessary. This potentially undermines the role of the pharmacist.

The supermarket model of consumerism (Winkler 1987) operates within pharmacies themselves as pharmacists control what is available, and thus, what may appear to be a choice of products is in practice restricted according to factors such as pharmacy policy or availability from, or 'special offers' by, suppliers.

The increasing availability of medicines may be seen as fuelled by the 'push' of government policy towards making people more self-reliant, as well as the 'pull' of the health-care consumer. These ideas are now examined in more detail in order to consider the possible impact of health-care consumerism on consultations between pharmacists and customers.

Consumerism

In the 1980s UK government policies demonstrated a marked preference for market mechanisms over state monopolies, thereby introducing the consumerist model to public services. The consumer now stands at the heart of New Labour's approach to the reform and modernisation of public services (Vidler and Clark 2005). Government action is seen as enabling and facilitating rather than resolving. Every citizen must now become an active partner in the drive for health, accepting responsibility for securing their own well-being (Rose 2001). This new 'will to health' is partially enabled through changes in health policy that recognise what are seen to be the increasing expectations of people. The importance of 'making sure that people can get medicines or pharmaceutical advice easily and, as far as possible, in a way, at a time and at a place of their choosing' is stressed (DoH 2000a). One way in which access to medicines has been increased is through the reclassification of a number of medicines from prescription to prescription free (DoH 2003b). The drive, therefore, is towards individuals adopting a self-reliant and commodified approach to health care.

The consumerist model assumes a knowledgeable and self-directing subject, capable of identifying and articulating individual wants as choices about services. Yet, there is a potential for mis-match between providers and consumers. Providers may not be ready for the consumer, believing themselves to be the location of knowledge or expertise. Alternatively, users may not be ready, or willing, to be consumers (Vidler and Clarke 2005).

Over a decade ago Fairhurst and May (1995) argued that the general climate pervading the UK National Health Service had encouraged patients to recognise themselves as consumers. The notion of the expert patient identified a shift in the location of expertise and raised questions about the relationship between the expert patient and the expert professional (Vidler and Clark 2005).

The 'asymmetry of knowledge' between medical practitioners and patients/consumers may be perceived as a major barrier to consumerism. Lupton (1997), based on her work on encounters between doctors and patients, suggested this was too simplistic, arguing that the major barrier was:

the almost unique nature of the medical encounter in relation to embodiment and emotional features. Dependency is a central feature of the illness experience and the medical encounter and serves to work against the full taking up of a consumer approach. (Lupton 1997: 379).

A similar point in relation to dependency by patients on health-care providers was made by Greener (2003). Yet, this does not mean that people necessarily reject the consumerist position, rather they may pursue both the ideal-type 'consumerist' and the 'passive patient' subject position simultaneously or variously, depending on the context (Lupton 1997).

Hibbert *et al.* (2002) identified and elaborated on a similar phenomenon in their discussion of pharmacy consumers' approach to the purchase of medicines, which they summarised as 'permissive' and 'challenging' consumer voices. These 'voices' were not identified with particular individuals; rather, a single person may express either view in response to differing circumstances. The permissive consumer perspective allowed a role for professional regulation in medicine sales. Consumers argued for caution in the wider availability of medicines and a need for surveillance. Challenging consumers were reluctant to be questioned, and generally felt they had sufficient knowledge through their existing experience. The focus here was on buying a product rather then obtaining a professional service. There appeared to be relatively little scope for a professional contribution in terms of tailoring the treatment to the individual consumer and giving individualised risk information.

Interestingly, Hibbert and colleagues (2002) suggested that the consumers in their study were not challenging the pharmacy staff's interventions because they felt they had an equivalent professional expertise. Rather, their challenge was based on questioning the relevance or usefulness of this expertise to their personal use of medicines. They concluded that consumerism represented a significant challenge to the accomplishment of medicines surveillance and professional work in the community pharmacy.

Pharmacy consumers may just want to complete what is essentially a commercial transaction promptly and efficiently (Bissell *et al.* 2000). In Bissell *et al.*'s (2001) study consumers stressed their ability to self-manage specific minor ailments using over-the-counter medicine. Such confidence stemmed in part from long-term personal experience of managing minor ailments successfully. Crucially, the majority of respondents expressed the belief that medicines available in the pharmacy must be safe, particularly medicines such as Nurofen, which are also available from general retail outlets. Finally, they contended that access to OTC medicine might provide people with a sense of autonomy over their own bodies.

Communication around OTC medicines is a complex process characterised by medical, retail and pharmaceutical discourses (Banks *et al.* 2007). It is important to remain cognisant that sales generally take place in a consumer environment in which sales of non-medical products such as cosmetics and beauty products are also made. This increases the potential for medicine sales to be perceived by consumers as indistinguishable from non-medicine purchases. There is also an underlying awareness on both sides that if a customer is not sold the medicine requested they can easily take their business elsewhere, leaving pharmacists particularly vulnerable to the effects of consumerism.

Government policy encourages public participation in consultations as well as a self-reliant and commodified approach to health care. The adoption of this in practice is, however, complex and is further complicated by community pharmacists' need to assert their professional position. We use a small-scale exploratory study conducted in two pharmacies in London to consider how professional expertise and consumer discourses in relation to the sale of OTC medicines are managed in practice.

Methods

Fieldwork

The pharmacies involved in the research differed from most pharmacies in certain key respects. The two joint owners of the two study pharmacies had developed a particular practice model focusing on increasing customer participation in consultations. The model was expressed both in the layout of the pharmacies and in the way consultations were conducted. Dummy boxes for pharmacy-only medicines were displayed on the shop floor.

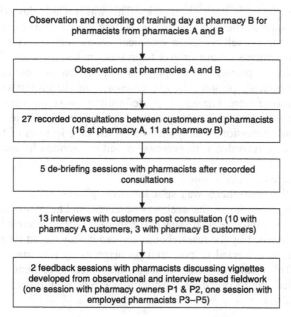

Figure 1 *Data sources.*

Consultations were conducted away from the counter, usually at the section appropriate to the presenting problem, the aim being to use dummy boxes of medicines as tools to aid an informed consultation. The pharmacy owners perceived this to be a crucial part of their practice model. Yet this is a notable departure from usual practice, as such medicines are generally kept behind the shop counter so that customers have visual access but cannot handle the medicines directly. Stock was restricted to 'health-related' items to create an environment focused on health without the distraction of products such as cosmetics and services such as photography. Moreover, the pharmacists themselves, rather than pharmacy assistants, led on consultations for OTC medicines, and together developed strategies for increasing participation by discussing cases drawn from practice.

The research project was set up as we were interested in how discussions about medicines were negotiated between customers and pharmacists, and the two pharmacy owners of the two study pharmacies were keen to have their model of practice examined specifically with regard to customers' reactions. Two Local Research Ethics Committees granted ethical approval.

This chapter draws on the following data: (i) an outline of the pharmacy owners' views of their practice model presented as part of a training day to the pharmacists they employed; (ii) data from observations and tape recorded consultations; (iii) interviews with customers and pharmacists about the interactions; and (iv) views expressed in two feedback sessions (one with the two pharmacy owners who led on implementing the practice model and the other with three of the pharmacists who worked in the pharmacies), discussing vignettes developed from observational and interview-based fieldwork in the two pharmacies. A chart outlining the data collection process is provided (Figure 1).

The training day
Fortuitously coinciding with the start of our project, the pharmacists who owned the pharmacies in which the fieldwork was to be conducted had organised a training day for

the pharmacists employed in both pharmacies. This was a whole day course that covered a number of areas such as the rationale behind setting up the pharmacies and the practice model subscribed to, as well as more technical issues such as systems of medicines management. Two members of our project team were invited to attend for an hour in the afternoon to explain our project and the practical implications of conducting the research. There were six pharmacists present, the two co-owners of the pharmacies and four other pharmacists who worked there. The session started with the two co-owners of the pharmacies presenting their views of their particular practice model. Then, following our brief presentation, there was some discussion, mainly focused on the practicalities of the fieldwork. The session was audio-tape recorded with permission and transcribed for analysis.

Observations and tape recorded consultations

The fieldwork in the pharmacies was split into two phases; initially, observations were conducted, ensuring every day of the week was observed, and fieldnotes written. In the next stage, people who came into the pharmacy and either showed an interest in or bought OTC medicine were approached by the researcher and asked if they would take part in the study. The researcher was also alerted to potential participants by pharmacy staff. In this way consultations for OTC medicines were identified and, subject to consent, were tape recorded and fully transcribed. We recorded 27 consultations (16 consultations from one pharmacy and 11 from the other).

Interviews with customers and pharmacists about the interactions

At the end of every recording day each pharmacist involved in a tape recorded consultation took part in a debriefing interview to examine their views of the recorded consultations they had taken part in that day.

We also recorded 13 semi-structured interviews with customers linked to 13 of the 27 recorded consultations (10 from one pharmacy and 3 from the other). Interviews focused on customers' views of the consultation they had recently had and their views of participation in consultations with pharmacists more generally. Customers were given the choice of location for the interview. Eight respondents chose to be interviewed in their own homes, three people worked rather than lived locally and were interviewed in their workplace, while two combined the interview with their weekly shopping trip and were interviewed in a café. Interviews varied in length between 15 and 40 minutes. There did not appear to be any difference in the length or quality of interviews at the different venues. All interviews with customers and staff were recorded and fully transcribed.

Feedback sessions

Two feedback sessions were held, one with the pharmacy owners (both of whom worked as pharmacists in the study pharmacies) and one with three pharmacists who worked in the pharmacies. The sessions consisted of general feedback and the presentation and discussion of vignettes developed from the observational and interview-based fieldwork. The aim was to gain pharmacists' overall reactions to the data. We constructed five vignettes that characterised the findings. These were: (i) customer wants a particular product and does not want to engage in any discussion; (ii) customer wants advice; (iii) pharmacist encourages participation and customer co-operates; (iv) pharmacist encourages participation and customer does not co-operate; and (v) pharmacist asks standardised questions with little attempt to tailor the interaction. The pharmacists were asked to read the vignettes and comment on each case in relation to the practice model favoured in the pharmacy and the reality of practice.

Setting
Both of the study pharmacies were in London. One was situated in a predominately middle-class area and attracted an older population. The other pharmacy was situated in an inner-city area, with a wider range of customers, including local minority ethnic groups as well as people who worked in the area. In this pharmacy, recruitment proved more challenging, particularly recruiting customers for interviews.

Analysis
The data were subject to a thematic analysis, with three members of the team reading all the transcripts and associated fieldnotes. Coding frameworks were independently developed. These were then discussed and merged in an analysis meeting. The resulting framework was refined in further meetings with all the project team as well as via electronic communication.

Here, we examine how professional expertise and consumer discourses in relation to the sale of OTC medicines are managed in practice. We initially consider data relating to (i) the participatory practice model advocated in the pharmacies under study; this is followed by findings relating to (ii) professional expertise; and (iii) consumer discourses.

The data
In the following illustrative extracts pharmacists are identified by the letter 'P' followed by a number, with P1 and P2 being used for the owners of the pharmacies. Customers are identified using the letter 'C' and a numeric identifier. Consultations are marked as 'C' at the end of the extract and debriefing sessions with pharmacists as 'debrief' followed by the consultation number to which the debrief refers. Interviews with customers are marked by the letter 'I'.

Results

The participatory practice model
Here, we outline the participatory model advocated by the pharmacy owners. This provides a context for considering potential congruence and conflict between professional expertise and consumer discourses in consultations for OTC medicines.

The pharmacy owners suggested that easy access to OTC medicines was vital for encouraging customer involvement. In their view, being able to 'actually pick up, touch, [and] look' (P1 – training day) at medicines facilitated customer participation. This was stressed in the initial training session in which they outlined their model and was reiterated in the feedback session.

In describing the layout of their pharmacies and access to dummy boxes of medicines the pharmacy owners talked about the 'defence' of the counter, suggesting that the counter operates both as a physical boundary between medicines and the public and to 'protect' the pharmacist. The practice model they advocated was designed to overcome both physical and interactional barriers.

In order to make the distinction between their model of practice and the model most commonly used in pharmacies, the pharmacy owners presented characterisations of the essence of the two types of consultation. In the first scenario the customer explained the problem and the pharmacist selected a medicine and directed the customer how to take it. This approach was summed up in the following way.

P1: You told us what's wrong with you. Now I know everything and I have been and done a whole lot of training and a whole lot of experience so I'm gonna reach down in this drawer behind the counter and I've chosen this for you and you have to take one three times a day (Training day).

This was contrasted with the second scenario, which was akin to their proposed practice model. Here, consultations are used to explore the customer's agenda and:

P1: their [the customer's] views of what the condition is and what medication they think they may need to help them (Training day).

They elaborated their approach by suggesting that providing customers with 'medical' options to describe their symptoms immediately closed down or limited the information exchanged.

P1: If someone comes up and says they've got a cough. Like you should, if you ask them; is it dry? Is it wet? That's not the right question.
P2: No you've already done it from a medical point of view, straight off haven't you? So they can only possibly have two coughs (Training day).

The practice model that was advocated aimed to facilitate the active involvement of customers in a discussion of their understanding of their problems and how medicines might help. In the training day, it was suggested that such an approach might prove particularly challenging for pharmacists as their training tends to endorse a structured approach to practice. In contrast, the approach advocated indicated the need for a more individualised approach to each customer, described as more like a conversation in which there might be some uncertainty about the exact direction it might take.

P1: It's a conversation really and you don't know quite where it's gonna go. And also you need some bit of skill to kind of direct it a bit (Training day).

The pharmacy owners struggled to explain exactly how their model could be operationalised, with one commenting that:

P1: It's very, suddenly now I realise, very hard to explain this even though we've been doing this for ages (Training day).

The model was developed incrementally through practice, hence the pharmacy owners' difficulties in articulating a clear process for operationalising the model. They perceived their approach to be innovative, particularly the incorporation of customers' views and preferences into decisions about medicines and the exclusion of non-health products in the pharmacies. They however felt unsure of customers' views of the model and how to judge success in relation to customer involvement, hence their participation in the research project.

The employed pharmacists did not appear confident in relation to the model. The training day did not include any discussion of stages of implementation, and they were expected to take the general description of the approach and incorporate it into their own practice, much as the pharmacy owners had done with their initial ideas. A request by one pharmacist for additional support in implementing the model was met with the reply that additional support was not necessary as they were already generally practising in this way.

Although the pharmacists might not have been clear about how exactly to operationalise the model, they were working in a pharmacy with a layout designed to encourage access to information about medicine via dummy boxes. They had also been exposed to the practice model via both the session that formed part of the training day and working alongside the pharmacy owners. The balance between professional expertise and consumer discourses was therefore likely to be different from that seen in other pharmacies.

Professional expertise

The model of practice advocated in the study pharmacies implied a shift in the relationship between pharmacists and customers. We consider both pharmacists' and customers' views of the role of professional expertise in order to examine potential openness to shifts in interactions in practice.

The practice model advocated combined pharmaceutical expertise with customers' beliefs, knowledge and preferences in an attempt to reach an agreed solution. Such an approach, however, cannot be taken to imply a lack of awareness on the part of pharmacists of an asymmetry of knowledge. The role and importance of professional knowledge was emphasised in relation to taking medicines safely.

> **P2:** It's about having an agreement with the patient as to what will happen *i.e.* they may be taking this medication it could be an OTC medication but you need to have an understanding of what will happen if medicine doesn't work or a side effect does happen (Training day).

When talking about the process of consultations one of the pharmacy owners commented on the potential need to correct or educate customers.

> **P1:** Because we're not trying to correct people necessarily. But it could involve some re-education (Training day).

The pharmacists emphasised the need for a balance between pharmaceutical expertise and the incorporation of the customer's perspective. It was however clear that in the event of a clash of perspectives pharmaceutical expertise took priority. Leading on from this, in one of the feedback sessions one pharmacist suggested that asymmetry of knowledge might act as a barrier to the development of a partnership between pharmacists and customers.

> **P3:** I was thinking about this thing about a negotiation between equals, that thing in concordance, and it's very hard when you're a medical professional and you do have more knowledge than patients to have an equal partnership (Feedback session with pharmacists).

Moreover, the pharmacists suggested that customers might consult them for advice and might not want to be involved in decision making despite the general rhetoric in society about involvement and participation.

> **P3:** Sometimes customers don't actually want the choice; they actually want to be told (little laugh) you know this is what you take and this will sort it out. If you start saying you should take this thing, or you could take that they get very erm confused. 'Oh which do you think?' Well I, you know . . . they're not used to having choices for everything. (Feedback session with pharmacists)

In this extract the pharmacist suggested that choice is not necessarily familiar in this context, despite general trends in wider society towards consumerism. This is in line with Lupton's (1997) work concerning the relationship between doctors and patients in which she suggested that the desire for dependency when ill may mean people may not adopt a consumerist role. In the following extract the pharmacy owners who promoted a model of participation talked of how customers may in practice resist this role. In their view, some customers came to the pharmacy for advice and did not expect to be involved in a discussion about that advice.

> **P2** . . . the patient they might think, 'I'm here for advice and this guy's asked enough!'
> **P1:** I think that actually is a very relevant point there. With the patient in the consultation sometimes I'm conscious of am I really stepping over the line and now hassling the patient for their understanding, because they've actually come, as you say, for good advice. (Feedback session with pharmacy owners)

Attempts to engage customers may in practice result in them feeling forced to respond. In the following example the customer had cystitis and looked to the pharmacist to advise her on which preparation to try. In the end, in an attempt to establish a basis for a decision, she asked about the popularity of sales, and took what was, somewhat reluctantly, suggested.

> **C:** What's the most popular? Is there a . . .
> **P:** Well. . . .
> **C:** Because I presume it's quite a . . . ?
> **P:** They're all . . . I just like that one because it's . . . well, it's got cranberries and cranberry is . . .
> **C:** Yeah, that's supposed to be good isn't it, for the . . .
> **P:** Cranberry is meant to be good as well, because that actually sort of the same thing.
> **C:** OK. Lovely.
> (C26 P2 C)

Even where customers were prepared to engage in a discussion about treatment, difficulties arose when they felt they had to express a preference for a particular treatment. This was particularly so if they did not have a clear basis for the preference yet their expressed preference appeared to be followed without question. This was evident in the following extract. The case concerned a mother who consulted on behalf of her eight-year-old daughter about suspected hayfever. When asked to express a preference she tentatively suggested her daughter might prefer an inhaler, but provided the caveat that her daughter did not really have any idea:

> **P:** What do you think you'd prefer at your place?
> **C:** Well she wanted an inhaler, that was her idea, but she's got no idea.
> **P:** Like a nose one? A nose one do you think?
> **C:** Er. Yeah.
> (C4 P1 C)

In the interview following the consultation, it transpired that the inhaler had not been used and the mother consequently questioned the basis for the inhaler being favoured over other options. No concerns were identified at the time of the original consultation; rather, concerns were triggered when there were problems with the medicine purchased.

Although the pharmacist presented other options, in line with the model of incorporating the customer's preferences, he had followed the mother's suggestion, despite the fact she did not seem totally sure. In the post-consultation interview it became clear that the mother felt the lack of direction given by the pharmacist was at least partially to blame for the failure of the treatment she purchased:

C: . . . I was looking for perhaps a nasal spray because that was the sort of thing I thought was supposed to be the most easy for her to take, because she's only eight years old.
[ ]
C: I felt that perhaps he could have questioned why I particularly wanted a nasal spray for the hay fever; perhaps he could have given me the other options and benefits, because the nasal spray, as it turned out, wasn't any good because my daughter wasn't happy using it. So I thought perhaps he could have given me the alternatives.
(C4 P1 I)

With respect to customers' expressions of their preferences in one of the debriefing interviews there was an interesting point raised about the pharmacist's possible ignorance about treatments. The pharmacist suggested she could not know everything and it was up to her to keep on learning so she could appreciate the points made by customers:

P4: . . . a lot of people read on the Internet of what they take things, and I have to say sometimes, even as a pharmacist, we're not, er, aware of what they're reading and what they're buying these things. . . . Because it was new to me that she was taking Acidophilus for irritable bowel syndrome . . . so it's something for me to learn and look up, obviously, you know.
(Debrief C 16/17)

This is an interesting comment as it suggested that the pharmacist perceived the onus to be on her to be informed so as to be able to comment on the information customers present in the consultation.

Pharmacists and customers both stressed the role and importance of pharmaceutical expertise. The other side to this is the extent to which customers presented themselves and pharmacists viewed them as consumers. Pharmacists' views of consumer discourses and the effect on consultations are considered next.

Consumer discourses
Pharmacists were aware customers have trusted sources of information outside the consultation and that these might be in direct conflict with the information they provide:

P1: Everything that we er speak about with the patient is actually going up in competition with what they already know. It might be what they already know from their next door neighbour who is a far greater source than us . . . if the next door neighbour told them something whether or not right medically they will stick with that (Training day).

In both of the feedback sessions there was a discussion of consumer discourses alongside the need to maintain the relationship with the customer. The following exchange demonstrates how views expressed by the customer might not be challenged or dismissed; even in the event they were not in keeping with the views of the pharmacist.

P: It looks like . . . it does look like an allergy, like an eczema type derma . . . what we call dermatitis, but I'd be really surprised if it was food related. Do you think it's food then?

C: I think I notice it whenever I eat eggs or chicken.

P: All right, well. All right, it must be then.

C: Well I don't know if I should be consulting my doctor on this.

P: Well, you'd still treat it the same way anyway, if it's caused by food or if it's caused by contact . . .

(C23 P2 C)

This may appear in contradiction to statements made earlier relating to the importance of pharmacists' expertise. However, as the treatment recommendation was not affected by the customer's view, rather than have an open disagreement the potential interactional problem was passed over and the topic switched from diagnosis to treatment.

The data presented here are in line with previous studies (*cf.* Hibbert *et al.* 2002, Lupton 1997) in suggesting that people may actively seek different types of consultation and levels of engagement depending on the presenting problem. Thus, customers spoke of visiting the study pharmacies specifically because of the level of information and advice provided:

C: that [the study pharmacy] is not the kind of chemist that you would go to if you . . . if I wanted a shampoo . . . But if I wanted to ask sort of information, medical information, I'd rather go to him, you know, rather than just go to some old pharmacy at one of the chains.

(C7 P1 I)

At other times people may view the pharmacy as a retail environment selling a particular product and do not want to engage in discussion or receive advice. This is demonstrated in the following extract. The customer had come in looking for something specific and was not interested in advice or any other products:

C: Before I had something like Hall's Menthalyptus. I don't want anything really kind of fancy, I just fancied . . .

P: Not a cough lozenge as such?

C: No, sorry . . . yes, just a cold type thing.

P: Just a . . . ?

C: I bought something here before, but I just couldn't . . .

P: Can I just bring you round here?

C: Yep.

P: I've got some Lockets, I've got some Soothers, but no Hall's at the moment.

C: You've got no Hall's? Oh, right!

P: I've got Soothers strawberry, and we've got Lockets.

C: No, I think I'll . . . I'll . . .

P: You want the Hall's?

C: I really wanted the Hall's because I find those much better than anything else. Only you haven't got any of those.

P: Have you tried anything like Fishermen's Friends?

C: Apparently they lower your potassium levels, my friend who's a nurse told me. *(laughs)*

P: OK.

(C25 P4 C)

The point here is that pharmacies may be used like any other shop to purchase a particular product. Pharmacists were aware of a tension between consumerism and their professional expertise. This tension was discussed in both of the feedback sessions, with an associated discussion of the strategies used, which generally involved selling the product requested.

P4: you just have to judge the ones who don't want, leave them and give them what they want, you know.
(Feedback session with pharmacists)

In some ways this fitted the preferred model outlined at the training day in that having had a discussion with a customer about a particular product the customer on the next occasion could just 'come directly to the counter and buy it' (P1 – Training day). Thus, the aim was informed customer choice not 'control' of access to medicines. The importance of the generation of repeat business was also noted, which of course was relevant in any decision to supply a requested medicine. Thus, both customers and pharmacists acknowledged the pharmacy to be a health-care *and* a commercial environment.

Discussion

This chapter has explored how pharmacists work to maintain their professional expertise while at the same time encouraging customers to participate in decisions about treatment. We focused on the use of over-the-counter medicines, considering the apparently contradictory concerns of professional expertise and consumerism, within the context of a particular model of pharmacy practice adopted in two pharmacies.

At first sight, the model of practice presented by the pharmacists, in line with the general trend towards encouraging partnership between pharmacists and customers, may be seen to indicate the need for a shift away from a reliance on pharmaceutical expertise in the consultation. However, in examining data from group discussions with the pharmacists (drawn from the presentation of the practice model as part of a training day and feedback groups with pharmacists), as well as observation data from practice and interviews with individual patients and pharmacists, this did not appear to be the case. There was no suggestion that attempts to engage customers in discussions about their treatment in any way necessitated a diminution of the importance of pharmaceutical expertise. Indeed, both pharmacists and customers acknowledged not just the existence but also the importance of the asymmetry of knowledge between pharmacists and customers. Pharmacists recognised, in line with Prior's (2003) point, that customers' knowledge may be inaccurate. Some customers appeared to lack the desire to exercise consumerist choice. Moreover, as has been noted elsewhere (*cf.* Wright 2004, Lupton 1997, Hibbert *et al.* 2002), making a choice in circumstances in which there appears no clear basis for the decision may be disempowering.

What was clear was the multiplicity of customer agendas. These varied from people who wished to purchase a medicine as they would any other commodity, to people who wished to discuss possible options, to those who wished to be told what to buy drawing on the pharmacist's professional expertise. This is in keeping with Hibbert *et al.*'s (2002) work on 'permissive' and 'challenging' consumer voices and Lupton's (1997) observations about patients adopting the 'consumerist' and 'passive patient' position in GP consultations simultaneously or variously, depending on the context. Yet, alongside an appreciation of pharmaceutical expertise, there was some discussion of consumerist behaviour. Pharmacists were aware that customers trusted sources of information outside the consultation, and of the potential interactional problems if views were expressed with which pharmacists disagreed. Moreover, there was evidence that customers actively chose a particular pharmacy depending on their need for advice.

The fact that the project focused on OTC sales in pharmacies is crucial in understanding the importance of customers' expressions of consumerism. Pharmacies, unlike other health-care settings, are also businesses. This has two main consequences; customers may treat pharmacies like any other consumer outlet, while pharmacists are likely to be sensitive to losing trade on both a single occasion and on any future ones. This is likely to have a major effect on interactions within the pharmacy and opportunities for the expression of pharmaceutical expertise.

The practice model described by the pharmacy owners may be seen to be rooted in both the health and commercial aspects of the pharmacies. The model aimed to encourage involvement in health and produce an agreed health-care solution, yet this solution should also provide a positive experience of health care and therefore encourage repeat business. There may however be a tension in relation to the practice model with respect to the use of dummy boxes. The pharmacists presented the use of dummy boxes as a way of informing customers and increasing access to information enabling choice, yet it is also possible to see this as a means of advertising pharmaceutical products. Moreover, it is important to remember that decisions about what to stock are made by pharmacists and, in line with the supermarket model of consumerism (Winkler 1987), choice is restricted according to factors such as pharmacy policy or availability from, or 'special offers' by, suppliers.

This chapter draws on a small data set, yet there was some discussion by pharmacists of the potential for disagreements due to customers' consumerist behaviour. We therefore conclude that further research using a larger dataset to investigate problems in interactions resulting from tensions between pharmaceutical expertise and consumerism is warranted.

References

Banks, J., Shaw, A. and Weiss, M.C. (2007) The community pharmacy and discursive complexity: a qualitative study of interaction between counter assistants and customers, *Health and Social Care in the Community*, 15, 313–21.

Bissell, P., Ward, P. and Noyce, P.R. (2000) Appropriateness measurement: application to advice-giving in community pharmacies, *Social Science and Medicine*, 51, 343–59.

Bissell, P., Ward, P. and Noyce, P.R. (2001) The dependent consumer: reflections on accounts of the risks of non-prescription medicines, *Health*, 5, 5–30.

Denzin, N.K. and Metlin, C.J. (1966) Incomplete professionalization: the case of pharmacy, *Social Forces*, 46, 375–81.

Department of Health (1996) *The NHS. A Service with Ambitions*. London: HMSO.

Department of Health (1999) *Patient and Public Involvement in the New NHS*. London: HMSO.

Department of Health (2000a) *Pharmacy in the Future – Implementing the NHS Plan*. London: HMSO.

Department of Health (2000b) *The NHS Plan – A Plan for Investment, a Plan for Reform*. London: Department of Health.

Department of Health (2001a) *The Expert Patient: A New Approach to Chronic Disease Management for the 21st Century*. London: Department of Health.

Department of Health (2001b) *Involving Patients and the Public in Health Care: Response to the Listening Exercise*. London: Department of Health (available at http://www.doh.gov.uk/involvingpatients/).

Department of Health (2001c) *Learning from Bristol: the Department of Health's Response to the Report of the Public Inquiry into Children's Heart Surgery at the Bristol Royal Infirmary 1984–1995* (Cm 5363). London: HMSO.

Department of Health (2003a) *The New NHS: Modern, Dependable.* London: HMSO.

Department of Health (2003b) *Building on the Best: Choice, Responsiveness and Equity in the NHS.* London: HMSO.

Department of Health (2005) *Choosing Health through Pharmacy. A Programme for Pharmaceutical Public Health 2005–2015.* London: HMSO.

Dingwall, R. and Wilson, E. (1995) Is pharmacy really an 'incomplete profession'? *Perspectives on Social Problems,* 7, 111–28.

Fairhurst, K. and May, C. (1995) Consumerism and the consultation: the doctor's view, *Family Practice,* 12, 389–91.

Greener, I. (2003) Patient choice in the NHS: the view from economic sociology, *Social Theory and Health,* 1, 72–89.

Harding, G. and Taylor, K. (1997) Responding to change: the case of community pharmacy in Great Britain, *Sociology of Health and Illness,* 19, 547–60.

Henwood, F., Wyatt, S., Hart, A. and Smith, J. (2003) 'Ignorance is bliss sometimes': constraints on the emergence of the 'informed patient' in the changing landscapes of health information, *Sociology of Health and Illness,* 25, 6, 589–607.

Hibbert, D., Bissell, P. and Ward, P.R. (2002) Consumerism and professional work in the community pharmacy, *Sociology of Health and Illness,* 24, 1, 46–65.

Lupton, D. (1997) Consumerism, reflexivity and the medical encounter, *Social Science and Medicine,* 45, 373–81.

Milewa, T., Dowswell, G. and Harrison, S. (2002) Partnership, power and the "new" politics of community participation in British health care, *Social Policy and Administration,* 36, 796–809.

National Pharmaceutical Association   (available   at   http://npa.journalistpresslounge.com/npa/ expertsissues/issues/index.cfm/fuseaction/details/id/EAFB87D0-13D3-97AA-2D6124ED95D86F70/ ses/1.cfm accessed 18 April 2007).

Newman, J. and Vidler, E. (2006) More than a matter of choice? Consumerism and the modernisation of health care. *Social Policy Review 18.* Bristol: Policy Press.

Nuffield Committee of Inquiry into Pharmacy (1986) *Pharmacy: a Report to the Nuffield Foundation.* London: The Nuffield Foundation.

Prior, L. (2003) Belief, knowledge and expertise: the emergence of the lay expert in medical sociology, *Sociology of Health and Illness,* 25, 3, 41–57.

Rose, N. (2001) The politics of life itself, *Theory, Culture and Society,* 18, 6, 1–30.

Vidler, E. and Clarke, J. (2005) Creating citizen consumers: New Labour and the remaking of public services, *Public Policy and Administration,* 20, 2, 19–37.

Winkler, F. (1987) Consumerism in health care: beyond the supermarket model, *Policy and Politics,* 15, 1, 1–8.

Wright, E.B., Holcombe, C. and Salmon, P. (2004) Doctors' communication of trust, care, and respect in breast cancer: qualitative study, *BMJ,* 328, 864–8.

9

In whose interest? Relationships between health consumer groups and the pharmaceutical industry in the UK
Kathryn Jones

Introduction

If ensuring the delivery of effective health care in modern welfare states requires a 'political settlement between important interests' (Moran 1999: 14), then it follows that, in balancing interests, policy makers must make trade-offs. For example political settlements to ensure the availability of safe and effective medicines must contend with the state's need to ensure access while containing costs, the medical profession's desire to maintain control over prescribing and the pharmaceutical industry's desire for profitability and a supportive research and development and regulatory environment. In other words, competing power relations play a formative part in the resulting health-care system. It also follows that any political settlement may need to be revisited as and when new pressures or agendas arise. Moran (1999) describes how in capitalist democracies, technological innovation may 'disrupt any equilibrium between [health-care] interests: it enriches some and impoverishes others' (1999: 14). He contends that the resulting competition may reshape political agendas, with both winning and losing interests resorting to the policy process to minimise damage and maximise benefits. Other pressures can also test agreements, for example changes in population demographics may increase strain on resources; or the arrival of new actors in the policy arena may challenge the long-held assumptions of existing interests (Baggott *et al.* 2005).

Indeed, policy making in health care, once the preserve of powerful interests, is now confronted by a hitherto inchoate voice, that of the health-care consumer (Baggott 2007, Salter 2004). Since the 1960s, health consumers have increasingly mobilised around particular medical conditions or in response to broader issues such as patients' rights. They have formed organisations to provide self-help, advice and advocacy. Health consumer groups – voluntary sector organisations that promote and/or represent the interests of patients, users and carers – (hereafter consumer groups[1]) reflect features of new social movements (Allsop *et al.* 2004). For example they are involved in confronting scientific knowledge with 'real world' experience; protesting against adverse events, and claim a representative role in policy making. Indeed, their perspectives on policy problems have been welcomed by established interests who have increasingly drawn on their expertise (Baggott *et al.* 2005). However, they lack the political and financial resources of other policy actors, and Lofgren (2004) cautions that their critical edge may be compromised through participation in governance structures and alliances with health professionals and industry.

These more powerful interests may simply be attempting to subvert the activities of consumer groups, reshaping or redefining their concerns to match their own, creating a situation which implicitly or explicitly mutes groups' critique of their actions. In other words, the agenda of the consumer group is 'captured', raising questions of independence, power and legitimacy. In the light of these concerns, the focus here is on understanding how UK consumer groups manage their relationships with one key interest in health care – the pharmaceutical industry. In addition, this chapter explores how these links affect broader policy debates around access to medicine, regulation of industry's promotional activities and the inclusion of consumer groups in policy deliberations.

Available evidence suggests that links between industry and consumer groups have grown recently (Baggott and Forster 2008, Ball *et al.* 2006). This, however, has given rise to fears that groups are being used by industry to indirectly lobby health-care decision makers, particularly in light of wider debates about the influence of the pharmaceutical industry over health-care delivery (Busfield 2006, Health Committee 2005, Health Action International 2002). A key concern is that groups may become too focused on securing pharmacological interventions for conditions which may be better served by alternative means (O'Donovan 2007). Indeed, in a recent survey, only 16 per cent of *bmj.com* readers agreed it was acceptable for groups to take industry funding (*British Medical Journal* 2007).

Yet, while their motives may differ, it is clear that industry and groups will share an agenda around the availability of, and access to, medicine. With globalised information networks, consumers can learn about treatments available in one health-care system and advocate their availability in another (Fox and Ward 2005). In the UK, the National Institute for Health and Clinical Excellence (NICE) has a key role in appraising the cost-effectiveness of medical technologies and in developing clinical guidelines on appropriate treatments. Its refusal to fund treatments, and delays in the implementation of NICE guidance, have done much to galvanise the activities of both industry and groups (Duckenfield and Rangnekar 2004). These actors may therefore simply be highlighting issues that other policy actors would rather remain hidden – cost constraints in the delivery of health care.

One difficulty in exploring the implications of collaboration is that groups are not required to disclose information on links with industry (Which? 2003). However, following revisions to the Code of Practice (ABPI 2005) which regulates the promotional activities of industry in the UK, the Association of the British Pharmaceutical Industry (ABPI) now requires companies to release this information on their websites or annual reports. This provides a useful baseline from which to determine acknowledgement of industry support and to make some judgements about the nature of the relationship. Drawing on broader ethical debates, however, it is recognised that disclosure of information is not a neutral phenomenon (Gray *et al.* 1996, Moon and Bonny 2001). Disclosure may reflect a desire for reputation management rather than a commitment to freedom of information (Gray *et al.* 1996). Nonetheless, a requirement for transparency provides access to information that would otherwise remain hidden, and it can reinforce openness by facilitating further demands for information (Gray *et al.* 1996). In the context of industry-professional relationships, Hurst and Mauron (2008) identify two key problems with disclosure: first, it may make any conflict of interest seem acceptable by appearing to legitimise activities, and second, acknowledgement of links may not be sufficient to assess the likelihood of bias. In this way disclosure may reflect and support existing power structures in society (Gray *et al.* 1996). Yet without public disclosure of the extent of contact, and the decision rules which underpin links, informed decisions about collaboration and influence are impossible (Ball *et al.* 2006, Jack 2006).

In exploring industry-group co-operation, this chapter addresses a number of key questions. How is collaboration and potential conflict of interest currently acknowledged? How are existing power relationships in the policy process affected by industry-group collaboration? Does collaboration with industry strengthen or undermine groups' legitimacy among policy makers? How should disclosure be regulated? The chapter is divided into three sections. The first provides an overview of positions taken by consumer groups on disclosing industry support, together with an assessment of the information provided on company and group websites. The second addresses both sectors' response to criticisms of organisational capture and the use of policies which outline how groups seek to manage links to industry. The final section addresses how other health-care stakeholders view these links and the wider policy response to issues of disclosure.

Methods

The chapter draws on a series of interviews with representatives of UK consumer groups, the pharmaceutical industry and other health-policy actors. They were undertaken in relation to two studies. The first, funded by the ESRC, on consumer groups in the UK health-policy process, was undertaken in three phases between 1999 and 2001 (Baggott *et al.* 2005). The initial phase entailed a semi-structured postal questionnaire sent to 187 groups (66% response rate (n = 123)). The second phase consisted of semi-structured interviews with leaders (chief executives and policy officers) from a sample of consumer groups (n = 39). The final phase involved semi-structured interviews with representatives (n = 31) from the health professions, government, Parliament, charities and ABPI (the UK drug industry's trade association). The second study, undertaken in 2005/6, was a pilot study of the pharmaceutical industry in the UK health-policy process (Jones 2007). Ten semi-structured interviews were undertaken with representatives (senior officers) from pharmaceutical companies and ABPI (n = 4), government (n = 3) and industry observers, including a consumer group (n = 3). In both studies, interviews were taped and transcribed. Using principles of qualitative data analysis, a coding framework based on multiple readings of interviews was devised and data were sorted into categories relating to internal and external relationships and sub-themes within these were identified. To maintain the anonymity of interviewees, respondents from the consumer group sector are referred to as 'CG', the pharmaceutical industry as 'PI' and government/stakeholders as 'GSH'.

The chapter also draws on an assessment in May 2007 of the Association of British Pharmaceutical Industry's full-members' websites detailing support given to consumer groups. Data were downloaded and recorded onto a matrix which logged group name, condition area, group type, and grant information. In some instances, companies also listed links with other health-care stakeholders,[2] such as professional associations and NHS trusts. These donations were however excluded from further analysis as the focus was on support for consumer groups. As a cross-check, the websites of consumer groups identified by industry were searched. Again, data were transposed onto a matrix which logged whether and how links were acknowledged. Websites were considered to be more up to date than annual reports, because of time-delays between submission to auditors and publication. In addition, websites of the 39 groups interviewed for the ESRC study were searched for up-to-date information on relationships with industry (following mergers and closures, 34 groups remained). This was undertaken as a check against change in circumstances to ensure that data from interviews were still valid.

Links between consumer groups and industry in the UK

This section explores disclosure by industry and consumer groups of links between the two sectors, it suggests three possible positions taken by groups on disclosure, and then compares and contrasts the level of detail provided by companies and groups. Not all groups seek to develop relationships with industry, some serve areas that may not require pharmacological intervention (*e.g.* natural childbirth). Other groups may represent those who have had adverse reactions to medication and have sought legal redress; again they are unlikely to accept links. The majority of groups, however, need to consider whether and how to collaborate with industry (Baggott *et al.* 2005). For their part, industry may seek links to gain access to groups' expertise, aid mutual understanding, raise public awareness of conditions and/or for altruistic reasons (Baggott *et al.* 2005). There have been a number of attempts to classify relationships that form between companies and other health-care stakeholders (*e.g.* Doran and colleagues (2006) on the medical profession; O'Donovan (2007) on consumer groups). In particular, distinctions are made between those who refuse links and the attitudes of those who accept them. Of interest here, however, is how consumer groups choose to disclose links with industry; evidence from the ESRC study indicates there are three possible positions:[3]

- Refusers: groups refusing contact with industry on principle, arguing it compromises independence, providing a definitive statement to this effect. It is likely that this position is adopted by a minority of groups; two of the 34 interview groups did so. For example, the National Heart Forum (2006) website states:
  'The NHF is an independent organisation and does not take money from commercial organisations or from the food, alcohol, tobacco, pharmaceutical or marketing industries. The NHF has limited resources in comparison to these industries and there is a need to constantly monitor industry practices. It is important to do this in an independent way that does not compromise the public interest.'
- Accepters: those accepting funding and/or links with industry; they however argue that any relationship should be transparent. These organisations have policies which guide their activities and make them publicly available. It is likely that this reflects a small but growing number of groups; nine of the 34 interview groups had policy guidelines. For example, one group interviewee said:
  We have an ethical policy round working with drugs companies . . . we will accept funding from drugs companies but as long as it doesn't have strings attached to it (CG38).
- Non-disclosers: groups that do not reveal details of acceptance or refusal of industry support. Twenty-three of 34 interview groups were in this category. However, it is likely that a significant number accept funding – eight interview groups were identified by a company as receiving support but did not acknowledge this themselves.

Industry support for consumer groups

Around 40 per cent of the Association of British Pharmaceutical Industry's 74 full-members listed financial and in-kind support for consumer groups on their websites. In total, industry provided 488 grants to 246 groups. Most companies (n = 15) listed between one and ten groups on their websites. However, as Table 1 below shows, nine companies, some of the largest in the sector, funded twenty or more groups with six disclosing additional information beyond group name.

It appears that industry is selective in the groups it supports, for example, the majority of groups (57%) were named by only one company, just over a quarter were named by two or three companies, and the remainder by four or more. Table 2 lists those groups named by six or more companies.

The company websites provided a varying amount of detail on links with groups. Less than half listed any information other than group name. Only 12 of the 29 websites noted the time-frame the agreements covered. While the majority of websites indicated that links

Table 1 *Pharmaceutical companies funding 20 or more consumer groups*

Pharmaceutical Company	Number of groups named	Disclosure of additional information	Profit reported in 2006* Million (USD)
Sanofi-aventis	68	No	10,359**
GlaxoSmithKline	60	Yes	15,972***
Pfizer	53	Yes	19,337
Janssen-Cilag	33	Yes	not available
Roche	32	No	8,143****
Bristol-Myers Squibb	32	Yes	1,585
AstraZeneca	22	Yes	6,063
Novartis	20	No	7,202
MSD	20	Yes	4,434

Source: Company Websites May 2007/*November 2007. **reported as 7,040 m Euros, ***reported as 7,808 m GB pounds, ****reported as 9,171 m Swiss francs.

Table 2 *Consumer groups named by six or more pharmaceutical companies*

Consumer group	Number of companies naming group
Cancerbackup	12
Diabetes UK	8
Blood Pressure Association	7
Men's Health Forum	6
National AIDS Map	6
National Rheumatoid Arthritis Society	6
Patients Association	6
Stroke Association	6

Source: Company Websites May 2007.

related to the provision of financial support, not all were explicit about the extent or purpose of funding. Only four companies (Bayer, GSK, Lilly and Co, and Pfizer) listed the amount provided to individual groups. Eight companies either made a general statement of why links were valuable or explained the purpose of specific grants. Three companies (GSK, Lilly and Co, and Pfizer) gave more comprehensive information and outlined principles governing their joint work, the amount and purpose of funding and the percentage of total income these grants accounted for. In addition, Astra Zeneca provided links to the formal agreements between it and named groups. Types of projects supported by industry ranged across sponsorship of conferences, publications, disease awareness campaigns, provision of core grants to cover groups' running costs, funding specialist nurses and/or research projects.

Of the four companies revealing the exact funding provided to groups, two-fifths of grants were for £9,999 or less, a quarter between £10,000 and £19,999 and 13 per cent between £20,000–£29,999. Only six per cent of grants were for £100,000 or more. The figures on percentage of funding provided by three companies showed that the majority of grants accounted for less than 10 per cent of total group income (31% of grants accounted for <1 per cent of income, 33% for 1–4.9 per cent of income, and 17% for 5–9.9 per cent of income). Significant contributions, where funding was over 20 per cent of total group

Table 3 *Conditions/areas receiving support from pharmaceutical companies*

Conditions/areas	Number of groups	%
Cancer	58	23
General Health	49	20
Mental Health	24	10
Neurological conditions	23	9
HIV/AIDS	21	9
Heart / Circulatory disease	17	7
Arthritis / related conditions	13	5
Other	41	17
Total	246	100

Source: Company Websites May 2007.
Other includes: diabetes, haemophilia and other blood disorders, infertility.

income, were provided in only nine per cent of cases. These figures suggest that concerns that industry 'bank-rolls' the consumer group sector are largely unfounded, although this assessment is based on data provided by those few companies providing sufficient detail to determine funding levels. Indeed, if more companies released this information, a more accurate assessment could be made. It appears, however, that the majority of groups are not reliant on the pharmaceutical sector for support.

Industry sponsored groups across a range of condition areas, summarised in Table 3. The majority of groups (23%) were concerned with cancers, either specific diseases or all cancers. Around 10 per cent of links were with groups dealing with mental health issues, neurological conditions or HIV/AIDs. Heart/circulatory disease and arthritis-related charities also attracted funding. This is unsurprising since these are major areas of drug research and therapy. A fifth of groups had a broader agenda rather than specific conditions, indicating that industry sees a role in supporting general issues such as patients' rights. The data also showed that around five per cent of groups were alliance organisations to which other consumer groups were affiliated.

Disclosure by consumer groups

A cross-check of consumer groups' websites revealed they were less likely than industry to acknowledge relationships. Only 26 per cent of groups known to receive industry support revealed this on their websites. While 10 per cent of groups did not have a website, nearly two-thirds gave no online financial information, although some provided access to annual reports which may acknowledge links (see Ball *et al.* 2006). The level of transparency and openness from those who acknowledged support also varied significantly. Four groups simply put the company's logo on their site, and three indicated that they accepted industry funding but did not identify where from. Twenty-two groups named individual companies and 18 gave details of the type of grant provided (mainly educational or unrestricted) and their purpose (for example, sponsoring websites, funding publications). Only 14 groups gave details of the financial arrangements, with four stating the percentage of income obtained. A similar number indicated they had policies for working with industry. In addition, a minority of groups gave no indication of links to industry, but provided details on their funding policy.

It is interesting to note that groups named most frequently by industry gave more details. Even so, a third gave no information. Of the 22 groups receiving grants from five or more companies, eight gave details of the policy governing these relationships and five listed the amount of funding received. Cancerbackup, which as noted earlier was listed by 12 companies, revealed the purpose and amount of funding, its policy on working with industry and the percentage of total income from industry. Overall, however, only a minority of groups disclosed links with industry, or set out a policy governing these relationships. Non-disclosure leaves the sector open to accusations of naivety at best and at worst, unprofessional or unethical conduct.

Managing the relationship

Rationale for links with industry
This section, from the perspective of groups and industry, explores why relationships between the sectors form and develop. It also examines how they view claims of conflict of interest that might arise from these links and the importance placed on ethical guidelines in structuring the relationship. Interviewees argued that, given their common agenda, communication between the two sectors was inevitable and relationships likely to occur. In part, it is a relationship between producer and consumer. For example, in its policy on working with industry, Cancerbackup argues:

> We believe it is important to maintain cooperative relationships with companies that manufacture and market cancer drugs . . . in order to foster communication between the patients Cancerbackup represents and the companies whose decisions will affect their treatment (Cancerbackup 2006: 1).

Groups were also pragmatic, arguing that without industry support some services they provided for the public would not exist (see also Baggott *et al.* 2005). For example, while acknowledging public concerns, the Stroke Association's respondent said:

> We recognise that, we know that and we work within those constraints, *i.e.* there are advantages to them but there are advantages to us because if a company is sponsoring a leaflet that costs, you know, £20,000 . . . that £20,000 can go somewhere else, either directly helping an individual that's had a stroke or perhaps funding new research.

Another interviewee whose organisation accepted sponsorship for a help-line argued that it remained independent and that accepting funding did not amount to support for industry products:

> Yes we do get criticised because it could be seen that there's a conflict of interest there. But they provide a resource for patients that wouldn't otherwise have that information. But we're not going to go out and flog their drugs for them (CG33).

Groups also argued that no funding source is dilemma-free, for example, the UK government's current emphasis on providing groups with project funding was linked to support for particular policies. Indeed, one group's website declared that it refused government funding because it would conflict with their policy-related activity.

Policy guidelines
The majority of groups were aware that industry had its own agenda, specifically the need to maximise profits, but argued that, despite this, it was possible to develop mechanisms to manage relationships. One interviewee said:

> Nobody should pretend that [company name] isn't driven by profit, but once you understand that then you can work out how you deal with it (CG40).

Mechanisms suggested by those endorsing links between industry and groups included policy guidelines which specify terms of reference for co-operation (Health Coalition Initiative 2005). Within the consumer group sector, calls for public disclosure have risen in recent years. In the late 1990s, the alliance organisation, Long-term Medical Conditions Alliance (LTCA) published *Working with the Pharmaceutical Industry: Guidelines for Voluntary Health Organisations on Developing a Policy* (Wilson 1998). A few years later, the UK consumers organisation, *Which?* published a critique of links between the two sectors (Which? 2003). This was a catalyst for some groups to produce their own policies or adopt others. For example, a small number of groups are signatories to *Health on the Net Foundation's* 'HonCode', which accredits good practice in the provision of online health information. Among its principles is disclosure of industry funding (HONF 2007). Policies serve both an internal and external role. The policies published by groups noted that their purpose was not just to inform companies of the ground rules for collaboration, but also to inform others about the nature of this relationship. For example, the Alzheimer's Society's (2006) policy states:

> The Society has prepared this note to help clarify what assistance it can and cannot give to pharmaceutical companies and those working for them and to define for interested parties its independence from the pharmaceutical industry.

The policies also noted internal decision rules for collaboration, often a statement that the Chief Executive must be persuaded the relationship would not bring adverse publicity or damage the charity's reputation. They also noted when the Board of Trustees – those responsible for ensuring compliance with charity law – would be involved in funding decisions. Yet, few stipulated the requirement for a written contract as advocated by the Long-term Medical Conditions Alliance guidelines (Wilson 1998). In addition to establishing decision rules, many policies outlined the principles underpinning relationships. For example, Arthritis Care (2005) listed: *transparency* – to ensure the relationship was not seen as an endorsement of the company or its products; *equal partnership* – working together to meet the needs of people with arthritis; *mutual benefit* – the relationship should benefit both parties; *independence* – ensuring the charity remained independent.

As would be expected, the policies discussed the management of financial arrangements. The majority suggested that groups would prefer any project to be funded by consortia of companies and that good practice required multi-source funding for projects. A number of policies noted members had the right of access to a range of interventions, not simply pharmacological. Policies were split between those that automatically disclosed funding and those that stated this was a matter of negotiation. One organisation stated the amount of funding would not be revealed unless the sponsoring company agreed, and two noted that only funding over £1,000 would be disclosed. Only one group noted the maximum funding it would accept in a given financial year.

Most policies stated the group would not endorse or promote industry's products (see also below). Groups also claimed full editorial independence: any publicity using their name or logo had to be pre-approved. Interviewees argued the value of these policies was to ensure an appropriate framework for co-operation and to guarantee transparency:

> The group had a pragmatic view of if you can get money out of people with no strings attached and you watch yourself very carefully and it's all very clear and written down in abundance then it doesn't really matter (CG11).

This point was acknowledged by industry interviewees. They suggested written policies and agreements were a useful tool for reputation management. In addition, they described how, given increasing public scrutiny, their own organisations had adopted more formal strategies for dealing with groups:

> At one stage work with patients' groups was viewed as a 'nice thing to do', and it wouldn't be looked at as part of pharmaceutical business interest. Now there is more scrutiny and scepticism of the industry, and corporate affairs work is an integral part of business (PC1).

A respondent from another company said:

> I think my view of why there has been an increased corporate focus is reputation management . . . [company name] got caught completely bank-rolling organisations and I think it's more to make sure that we are behaving appropriately, that there is more corporate control (PC2).

Ethical issues: A political alliance?
Consumer groups argued that while collaboration may accrue differential benefits, theirs was an equal partnership. In addition, there were areas where both sectors had similar concerns, for example, in publicising conditions and ensuring access to treatment, as one group interviewee said:

> We both share a number of objectives and one is to get arthritis higher up the political agenda and another is to get the general public more aware of arthritis and another is to try to empower patients because all three of those things are in our mutual interest. What we try and do is find ways of working that achieve those benefits for most of us (CG17).

A few group representatives suggested their influence and involvement in the policy process meant industry had an interest in ensuring their success. Offering support for member-based activities could free-up resources for lobbying, it was argued, to the benefit of both parties. A representative of an alliance group said:

> I would say the influence of patients' groups in most views is far higher than that of the pharmaceutical industry. And that might be why the pharmaceutical industry wants a relationship with patients' groups because it sees them succeeding in achieving their objectives as being useful to the pharmaceutical industry (CG40).

However, groups were wary of working too closely with industry on policy issues, believing it would damage their credibility; concerns about perceived impropriety were paramount. For example, a mental-health group, which had audited access to new generations of anti-psychotic drugs, said that had the audit been sponsored by a company, policy makers would assume bias: 'you could argue until you are blue in your face that it had been independent . . . (but) it wouldn't matter' (CG23). Some group websites stressed that industry funding was not used for lobbying purposes. For example, the Alzheimer's Society which sought a judicial review on NICE's rejection of three drugs to treat early-stage dementia, publicly stated that industry funding was not used for campaign activity (Alzheimer's Society 2006).

Respondents from industry agreed that they shared a common agenda with groups, and that groups were increasingly influential policy actors. One company respondent explained why links were important: 'they do want access to medicines, so if they have a voice that helps us . . . It's in our interests for patients' groups to have a reasonable voice' (PC2). Given that groups lobby for access to optimum care, companies undoubtedly benefit from another voice making similar demands. Yet in response to criticisms that funding of member-based activities amounts to undue influence, industry representatives argued that groups place a premium on their independence, taking a lead role in any relationship:

> They are professional organisations who are independent and capable of advocating on their own terms, the corollary of that is they do not want to be seen as anyone's poodle . . . It's no longer a question of industry being able to advise how or what particular issues to proceed with, it's very much done on NGOs' terms (PC3).

Ethical issues: promoting industry products?

Given the reliance on pharmacological intervention in medical care, it is inevitable that groups develop views on specific drugs, particularly newer treatments which may have more potential for improving quality of life. A core concern for groups was how to approach this, while concurrently managing links with industry. In interview, the majority of groups were aware of accusations of promoting company products, although one interviewee suggested claims about endorsement are over-stated:

> Patients, you have to remember, aren't necessarily always aware which company produces the drug if they just take them, so the drug companies who put their name on our literature, our patient doesn't know which drugs they produce . . . so I can't see how on earth can there be any ethical problems (CG39).

With the growing focus on evidence-based health care and in particular the advent of NICE guidance, groups face new dilemmas about endorsing products. For example a breast cancer alliance representative stated: 'if we're campaigning for equality of access to the best then there's going to be times when we're campaigning for equality of access to a specific drug' (CG36). Indeed, the public's right to access best-practice treatment was noted in various policies, for example, Cancerbackup's (2006: 1) policy states:

> Cancerbackup does not endorse individual treatments of whatever kind . . . however, if there is widespread consensus that a particular type of treatment might be beneficial for cancer patients, if for example it has been recommended by the NICE, then the charity has no hesitation in calling for funders to make resources available to implement NICE guidance.

Dilemmas over industry funding also arise when concerns about drug safety and efficacy are raised. In 2005, various arthritis charities, including Arthritis Care, were criticised for accepting funding from the manufacturer of rofecoxib, withdrawn from the market due to safety concerns (Frith 2005). In response, Arthritis Care (2006) pointed to its ethical guidelines, noted that the company had provided less than one per cent of its total income in 2003/4, and highlighted how it publicised concerns about the drug to its members. Clearly, it is difficult to balance the tension between maintaining co-operative relationships and criticising industry. The mere accusation of impropriety may damage a charity's reputation irrespective of any policy to which it is committed.

The views of stakeholders and policy developments

So far, the chapter has explored the extent of contact between industry and consumer groups. It has argued that although policy guidelines are recommended, the majority of groups have not publicly adopted them. This section examines how other policy actors view industry-group collaboration, particularly around issues of influence and transparency. It then explores how criticisms relating to disclosure have brought a regulatory response from within and outside industry. Stakeholders have accepted there would be links between the two sectors, noting their shared interests. However, they have also suggested that there were pragmatic reasons why industry would seek collaboration. For example, one interviewee said:

> The difficulty for the industry is that a cynic might just say 'you are just in it for the money aren't you?', so it's in their interest to get third-party endorsement from something like a charity or a patient group or a body with medical expertise or kudos to give it a bit more credibility, and you can sort of understand why that would be the case (GSH6).

Others argued as long as there was public disclosure about links, then policy makers should not be too concerned. A Department of Health civil servant noted:

> Each group has a responsibility to their shareholders/stakeholders to do the best for their organisation and in some cases that is to lobby government, get your point across; so long as that is done in an open and transparent way and everyone understands the relationships that's all right, I'm not clear that's always been the case . . . (GSH5).

Indeed, the transparency of industry's relationships with other policy actors was one focus of the recent UK Parliamentary Health Committee's investigation into the influence of the pharmaceutical industry (Health Committee 2005). At the time, industry was concerned with the committee's agenda as a number of its advisors were known critics of industry practices (Jones 2007). As part of its remit, the committee addressed links between industry and consumer groups, and while it recognised that there were reasons for co-operation, it was critical of non-disclosure, recommending that:

> Patient groups be required to declare all substantial sources of funding including support given in-kind and make such declarations accessible to the public (Health Committee 2005: 119).

Around the same time the Association of British Pharmaceutical Industry reviewed its Code of Practice for industry's promotional activities (ABPI 2005). Previously, it had not explicitly addressed relationships with consumer groups. The revised version, however, gives clear guidance, requiring companies to declare publicly which groups they support, and have a written agreement outlining terms of reference. Interviewees from both groups and industry suggested that increased scrutiny from policy makers prompted stronger guidance, the ABPI preferring to maintain self-regulation rather than risk a statutory response.

Government has also chosen to promote self-regulation to improve disclosure by consumer groups, rather than pursue amendments to charity law (Department of Health 2005). An interviewee noted:

> Post (health committee) report there is a very big sensitivity about the issue . . . I do think the industry is going to be a lot more careful. Probably patient organisations are as well . . . I think groups will get a lot better at declaring their relationships and so on (CG40).

Discussion

This chapter has examined how and why consumer groups and pharmaceutical companies disclose information on their financial relationships. It has shown that while concerns have consistently been raised about the nature and effects of these links within the context of a regulatory process which now requires disclosure from one party (industry) and recommends disclosure by another (consumer groups), a lack of transparency still persists. This lack of disclosure makes it difficult to fully assess the consequences of such links for the policy process; however, some tentative conclusions may be drawn.

Consumer groups share policy concerns with industry specifically around the profile of particular conditions and access to medication. It is no surprise therefore that they explore avenues where they have mutual interests. Indeed, across both studies, interviewees accepted the likelihood of this, although they also argued groups and industry should recognise potential conflicts of interest. These links have evolved at a time when the state has developed new regulatory processes for the approval of drugs and the development of treatment guidelines. This has had the potential to disrupt what Moran (1999) terms the 'political settlement' between state and industry around markets for industry products. Evidence from this study shows that consumer groups claim an interest in these policy debates and have at times increased pressure on the state to overturn NICE rulings.

So has industry captured the policy agenda of UK consumer groups in these debates? The findings presented here suggest not. It is unsurprising that groups insist on the availability of drugs which in their view prolong or improve quality of life. Consequently, they may question, critique and challenge government decisions to restrict or refuse funding for treatments they believe would benefit their members. From the perspective of groups, that this mirrors industry's agenda is a secondary consideration, and while industry representatives recognised they benefited from consumer groups holding other health-care stakeholders to account, they were adamant that they remained independent. Gauging whether groups are more concerned with the availability of drugs at the expense of other interventions is more problematic. Only a small number of funding policies commented on the rights of patients to pursue a range of treatment options. This said, consumer groups pursue a broad agenda in the policy process beyond the availability of drugs, adopting a holistic view of the needs of patients, users and carers (Baggott et al. 2005). In addition, it should be noted that groups, including those accepting funding, also use the policy process to hold industry to account, for example around adverse pharmacological reactions.

It is also unlikely that the interests of groups have been captured due to dependence on industry resources. While industry clearly supports a range of groups across a number of conditions, the evidence from websites (albeit limited) suggests it is not systematically bank-rolling the UK consumer group sector; in most cases funding from industry is only a small proportion of a group's total income. Where industry has supported the formation of a small number of groups, this has not necessarily been done in a clandestine way

(Baggott *et al.* 2005), although that it has identified a gap in provision is noteworthy. Funding from industry for member-based activity, may free up resources for groups to pursue their policy goals; however, as already stated these may or may not reflect those of industry. If industry funding was withdrawn, it is highly unlikely that groups would be forced to cease participation in the policy process.

Finally, does disclosure reduce or reinforce concerns about power imbalances? Currently, the lack of systematic disclosure by both sectors suggests that unease about the nature of links will endure. Their *shallow* approach to transparency simply strengthens critiques of undue influence because the necessary detail to facilitate informed decisions is withheld. This lends weight to those who suggest that a move to regulate disclosure is an attempt to capture the agenda of those who believe such relationships are inherently problematic (Gray *et al.* 1996, Hurst and Mauron 2008). Properly executed disclosure, however, can challenge these critiques. If the good practice adopted by some was replicated across both sectors, informed decisions about the implications of collaboration could be made (Gray *et al.* 1996). Given the role claimed by consumer groups as representatives of the public interest, it is important they acknowledge sources of funding. While there are pockets of good practice, and some relationships are becoming increasingly structured through codes of conduct and explicit statements of intent, the lack of disclosure about funding sources from the majority of groups suggests this may ultimately reduce the willingness of policy makers and other health-care stakeholders to see them as the legitimate voice of patients, users and carers in the policy process.

Notes

1   It is recognised that the term 'health consumer' is contested. However, 'health consumer group' accommodates the broad nature of citizens' interactions with the health-care state (for further discussion see Baggott *et al.* 2005).
2   Industry websites listed 57 grants to 54 health-care stakeholder organisations.
3   Figures add up to 34. Five groups had merged or closed since 2001, one did not have a website.

References

ABPI (2005) *Code of Practice for the Pharmaceutical Industry*. London: Association of British Pharmaceutical Industry.
Allsop, J., Jones, K. and Baggott, R. (2004) Health consumer groups in the UK: a new social movement? *Sociology of Health and Illness*, 26, 6, 737–56.
Alzheimer's Society (2006) Relationship with pharmaceutical companies, (www) www.alzheimers.org.uk (Accessed May 2007).
Arthritis Care (2005) Arthritis Care corporate sponsorship policy (available at www.arthritiscare.org.uk, accessed May 2007).
Arthritis Care (2006) Arthritis Care statement on Vioxx, (www) www.arthritiscare.org.uk (Accessed May 2007).
Ball, D., Tisocki, K. and Herxheimer, A. (2006) Advertising and disclosure of funding on patient organisation websites, *BMC Public Health*, 6, 201.
Baggott, R. (2007) *Understanding Health Policy*. Bristol: Policy Press.
Baggott, R. and Forster, R. (2008) Health consumer and patients' organizations in Europe, *Health Expectations*, 11, 1, 85–94.
Baggott, R., Allsop, J. and Jones, K. (2005) *Speaking for Patients and Carers*. Basingstoke: Palgrave.

BMJ (2007) Should patient groups accept money from drug companies? (www) http://resources.bmj.com/ bmj/interactive/polls/accept-money-poll (Accessed May 2007).

Busfield, J. (2006) Pills, power, people: sociological understandings of the pharmaceutical industry, *Sociology*, 40, 297–314.

Cancerbackup (2006) Cancerbackup policy and guidelines on working with pharmaceutical companies (available at www.cancerbackup.org.uk, accessed May 2007).

Department of Health (2005) *Government Response to the Health Committee's Report on the Influence of the Pharmaceutical Industry* (Cm 6655). London: DH.

Doran, E., Kerridge, I., McNeill, P. and Henry, D. (2006) Empirical uncertainty and moral contest: a qualitative analysis of the relationship between medical specialists and the pharmaceutical industry in Australia, *Social Science and Medicine*, 62, 1510–19.

Duckenfield, M. and Rangnekar, D. (2004) *Patient Groups and the Drug Development Process*. London: UCL.

Fox, N. and Ward, K. (2005) Globalised consumption and the challenge to pharmaceutical governance, *British Medical Journal*, 331, 40–2.

Frith, M. (2005) Exposed: Vioxx firm's cash payments made to arthritis charities, *The Independent*, 24 August.

Gray, R., Owen, D. and Adams, C. (1996) *Accounting and Accountability: Changes and Challenges in Corporate Social and Environmental Reporting*. London: Prentice-Hall.

Health Action International (2002) *Patients' Groups and Industry Funding*. Netherlands: HAI.

Health Coalition Initiative (2005) *A Framework Document for Developing Partnerships between VHOs and the Pharmaceutical Industry*. London: HCI.

Health Committee (2005) *The Influence of the Pharmaceutical Industry, HC 42-I*. London: TSO.

HONF (2007) HonCode accreditation system, (available at www.hon.ch, accessed May 2007).

Hurst, S.A. and Mauron A. (2008) A question of method: the ethics of managing conflicts of interest, *EMBO Reports*, 9, 2, 119–23.

Jack, A. (2006) Too close for comfort? *British Medical Journal*, 333, 13.

Jones, K. (2007) Pharmaceutical policy in the UK. In Hann, A. (ed.) *Health Policy and Politics*, 2nd Edition. London: Ashgate.

Lofgren, H. (2004) Pharmaceuticals and the consumer movement: the ambivalences of 'patient power', *Australian Health Review*, 28, 2, 228–37.

Moon, C. and Bonny, C. (eds) (2001) *Business Ethics*. London: Economist Books.

Moran, M. (1999) *Governing the Healthcare State*. Manchester: MUP.

National Heart Forum (2006) Supporting the NHF (available at www.heartforum.org.uk, accessed May 2007).

O'Donovan, O. (2007) Corporate colonization of health activism? Irish health advocacy organizations' modes of engagement with pharmaceutical corporations, *International Journal of Health Services*, 4, 37, 711–33.

Salter, B. (2004) *The New Politics of Medicine*. Basingstoke: Palgrave.

Which? (2003) Who's injecting the cash?, *Which?*, (April), 24–5.

Wilson, J. (1998) *Working with the Pharmaceutical Industry*. London: LMCA.

10

The great ambivalence: factors likely to affect service user and public acceptability of the pharmacogenomics of antidepressant medication

Michael Barr and Diana Rose

Introduction

The prevalence and virulence of depressive disorders are well established. It is estimated, for instance, that at least one in five persons will suffer from depression at some point in their lives (Solomon 2002). By 2020 the World Health Organization approximates that depression will account for nearly six per cent of the global disease burden and will rank second only to ischaemic heart disease as the leading cause of years lost to disability (WHO 2001).

Given the increasing diagnosis of depression, it is not surprising that the use of antidepressant medication has risen sharply in recent years.[1] In the United States, antidepressant use has tripled in the last decade. It is estimated that one out of every ten women in the US is taking an antidepressant (Vedantam 2004). In England, 8.2 million prescriptions were dispensed in 1999; four years later, this figure had jumped to over 19 million (MHRA 2004). Yet with more than a dozen different types of antidepressants on licence, there still exists no clear criterion for practitioners to know which drug to give to which patient. Thus, physicians often rely on guesswork and personal preference when prescribing. There is no guesswork, however, as to the profits involved. The drug Prozac alone has earned $2.6 billion annually for its manufacturers Eli Lilly and Company. In total; the European market for psychotropic drugs reached $4,741 million in 2000 (Rose 2005).

Despite their widespread use, there are significant problems with antidepressants. Approximately 40 per cent of people who take them receive no therapeutic benefit. Even when a patient does respond to a particular type of antidepressant, there are often considerable adverse drug reactions, which often lead people to discontinue use, since the therapeutic benefit takes several weeks to begin but the side effects are immediate. Many patients report that the trial and error process of finding an antidepressant that works can often add to their anxiety and suffering.

The promise of pharmacogenomics

Given the pervasiveness of depression and the profitability of antidepressants, it is not hard to see why such drugs are an attractive target for pharmacogenomics – that is, for research which aims to understand better the genetic variations in the metabolic enzymes (in the case of many antidepressants thought to be CYP2D6 and CYP2C19), transporter genes, proteins, and carriers that contribute to antidepressant adverse drug reactions (ADRs). Whilst there is no dominant model as to how pharmacogenomics is, or will, be, adopted in a clinical setting, it is clear at least that progress is slow and uneven[2] (Martin et al. 2006). Even when pharmacogenomics is at its best, information derived from tests is probabilistic and relative, not deterministic, providing help for prescribing physicians and their patients, but no patent solutions (Lindpaintner 2002).

Genome-based therapies for depression (GENDEP)

In this chapter we aim to explore the range of factors that may impinge upon public and service user acceptability of the pharmacogenomics of antidepressants. We relate these findings both to clinical and sociological literature on depression and antidepressant medication, as well as to broader discussions regarding the development of pharmacogenomics as a promissory technology. We conclude that the uptake of genome-based therapies for depression cannot be separated from wider issues regarding the meanings of mental illness and the significance of taking drugs that have moods as their targets.

The project from which this chapter originates formed the ELSI (Ethical, Legal and Social Issues) agenda of a study funded by the European Commission known as Genome-based therapies for depression (GENDEP), whose aim was to identify genetic variations that may affect responses to antidepressants. GENDEP was a three-year grant, begun in 2004, that aimed to recruit 1,000 depressed patients across eight European countries (England, Poland, Slovenia, Italy, Belgium, Denmark, Germany, and Croatia). To be included in the study, participants must have been diagnosed with at least moderate depression according to ICD-10 or DSM-IV criteria; aged 18–65; of either gender and of white ethnicity with European parentage. GENDEP excluded pregnant women, patients with a history of bipolar affective disorder or schizophrenia in first-degree relatives, as well as patients with substance abuse, primary organic disease, or treatment failure with one of the two antidepressants used in the study, Escitalopram or Nortripyline.

GENDEP participants were recruited through GP clinics or psychiatric care units. Researchers took DNA samples via blood, and attempted to correlate a patient's genetic information with their response to whichever study drugs the patient had been placed on. To make correlations between drug response and genetic make-up, GENDEP participants underwent a series of interviews and questionnaires to ascertain how they were feeling and to what degree they were experiencing side effects. Thus, patient volunteers received weekly phone calls and had several face-to-face meetings with GENDEP staff. The questionnaires were extensive and included the HAM-D, the Beck Depression Inventory, the Global Assessment Scale, MADRS, the UKU side-effects check-list, and a sexual functioning questionnaire. After 12 weeks, patients were discharged from the study and returned to the care of their original physician or psychiatrist.

Methods

In seeking to investigate both general public and mental health service user views regarding the acceptability of the pharmacogenomics of depression, we held a series of focus groups in four European countries associated with the GENDEP study.[3]

General public focus groups

We organised a series of focus groups with members of the general public in: London, England; Poznan, Poland; Aarhus, Denmark; and Berlin, Germany. Each site held three groups with a random sample of eight participants each. Participants were of mixed gender, ethnicity and age. Participants in Denmark and Germany were recruited via public adverts in local newspapers and magazines. Participants in England and Poland were recruited through a social science marketing agency. Exclusion criteria were anyone with direct experience of depression or antidepressant medication. All group members were paid £25 or its equivalent to compensate for their time and travel costs.

A facilitation guide was developed with the aid of literature reviews. The guide was tested via two pilot focus groups with university students in London. All facilitation materials and consent forms were translated from English into the relevant language. Facilitators from Denmark and Poland attended the groups in London to observe our aims and methods.

We travelled to Germany to assist with the organisation of the groups there. All facilitators were native speakers in the language in which the groups were conducted.

In addition to these focus groups, we also organised a half-day workshop (in London only) with recognised experts to discuss the policy-related implications of pharmacogenomics. Attendees included representatives from mental health charities, the pharmaceutical industry, academia, and psychiatry. Discussion was taped and transcribed.

Service user focus groups

The service user focus groups were conducted by researchers from the Service User Research Enterprise (SURE) at the Institute of Psychiatry in London. SURE conducts research from the service user perspective and is staffed mostly by people who are using or have used mental health services. In accordance with this, the service user focus groups in our study were facilitated by service user researchers.

Service user group participants were recruited through user organisations in each country. In Germany and England, participants were recruited consequent upon a survey which asked respondents whether they would take a pharmacogenomic test. In Poland, the participants were recruited direct via the national service user organisation.

The team experienced great difficulty in this recruitment process. One service user organisation in England refused to be part of the study because it dealt with pharmacology and genetics, two ideas that they objected to in principle. In Germany, recruitment was again difficult and laborious. The Board of the German user organisation initially refused to take part in the study but later relented on condition that the SURE researcher attend the group's assembly and present our project aims. At the assembly, our researcher met many objections but it was finally agreed that the research could proceed, an outcome which we partly attribute to the fact that she was well known to the group beforehand. The service user organisation in Denmark has, to date, refused to allow the research to go forward despite more than two years of contact. Again, we attribute this resistance to a rejection of the very principle of pharmacogenomics on behalf of the survivor/user movement.

As responses to the survey in England and Germany indicated high levels of agreement with pharmacogenomics, we became concerned that given the problems cited above with recruitment, our focus group findings might have been biased towards those with positive opinions. For example, in the English groups, responses might have been less supportive if the service user organisation opposed to genetic research had agreed to participate in our groups. We therefore recruited a group of users in Germany who had not completed the survey to ascertain why. We also ran a focus group with Board members of the pan-European user/survivor organisation European Network of (ex) Users and Survivors of Psychiatry (ENUSP). By using these methods of recruitment we hoped to provide a more balanced picture.[4]

Both public and service user group meetings lasted approximately two hours. Facilitation included an initial introduction to the pharmacogenomics of depression and then a series of prompts designed to get participants talking in general terms about the topic. The second half of public groups used two vignettes to elicit participant views on the main research questions of the study. Tapes were transcribed in their native language, then translated into English.

Analysis

The team worked together during the coding phase to explore key themes and categories in the data. This phase of data analysis helped establish the validity of categories and identify analytical themes. We used action-oriented sequential analysis when appropriate and where quality of the transcription permitted, in order to help provide a wider context for the discussion, group norms, and the processes by which respondents replied. (Kitzinger 1994; Wilkinson 2005). Thematic analysis was supported by NVivo 2. Initial categories were drawn from the topic guide. These were applied to see how far they captured the meanings in the texts. Further themes emerged on re-reading the transcripts and these were added to the coding frame. This process of iteration was repeated until theoretical saturation was reached (Silverman 2000).

Reflexivity in the research process: contributing to expectations
Like other biotechnologies that promise medical breakthroughs, pharmacogenomics is a 'promissory technology', built on the expectation that present research will reap future benefits. But since pharmacogenomics testing for depression is not at present a clinical reality, we faced the problem of having to simultaneously introduce the topic to respondents whilst asking their views on it. Inevitably, how we presented pharmacogenomics and our own beliefs regarding the technology will have impacted on the findings. There is some evidence, for example, that service users are more comfortable and more willing to take a critical stance when being interviewed by a service user researcher (Clark *et al.* 1999, Rose *et al.* 2003). In our presentation of pharmacogenomics, we tried to maintain a balance by explaining that GENDEP researchers were 'exploring the genetic factors that are suspected to be involved in the metabolism of antidepressant medications', and that 'some people hope that understanding how genetic make-up can affect drug response will result in greater antidepressant efficacy, allowing physicians to prescribe drugs that have fewer adverse reactions'. In the latter half of group discussions, we used case-based vignettes to help us explore some of the ethical issues around pharmacogenomics, such as orphan medicines, racial stratification, and drug access. We amended the cases as appropriate to take into consideration differences between the sites' various health care delivery systems.

In the course of conducting a large trans-national study such as this, it is possible to forget that we are not merely responding to the consequences of a technology but rather, are playing an active role in contributing to the production of hope surrounding the possible success of that technology (Hedgecoe and Martin 2003). Brown (2003) reminds us to be alert to the 'situatedness of expectations' and the role that hype can play in helping to legitimate research agendas to various publics. Indeed, it is the hitherto unfulfilled promise of pharmacogenomics which provided the rationale for the funding of GENDEP. Research such as ours can however plausibly cut both ways – that is, it may serve to help create a vision that mobilises patients to support a promissory technology, and/or it could help define the limits of the technology in terms of its public acceptability.

We note that at times our data are as much about depression and antidepressants as they are about pharmacogenomics. In part this may be a reflection of the fact that people are most comfortable talking about what they know best and, for reasons we have just described, this was not pharmacogenomics. We did attempt to keep discussion focused on pharmacogenomics as much as possible until it became clear that the desire to talk about the wider issues (the significance of an illness and the meanings of medication) was an important finding with implications for the acceptability of genome-based therapies.

Data and discussion

Analysis yielded several clear analytical themes which we describe below. These include general views regarding the acceptability of pharmacogenomics and findings which illustrate how wider perceptions of depression, antidepressants, and genetic research may impact on the reception of genome-based therapies.

Views on the pharmacogenomics of depression
One limit of our study is that we lacked the time and resources to make extensive trans-national comparisons. This would have required in-depth analysis of national and local variations in the four sites of respective health care systems and mental health services. In general terms, however, we make several observations. First, a majority of participants in all the public focus groups felt that pharmacogenomics was a 'good idea', felt 'positive towards it' and, in one case at least, would 'have it straightaway'. However, it is clear from our data that support was strongest in Poland where every participant in every group voiced support for the technology, and were on the whole less critical than other sites. Whilst it is possible, of course, that members may have been reluctant to deviate from majority opinion in a group setting, data clearly indicate that the Polish groups saw genetic technology as 'futuristic' and largely unproblematic. It is likely that the current state of mental health care in Poland influenced group members. For example, we were told by group members that in Poland antidepressants are relatively expensive compared to other countries. In addition, according to one study, Poland has the longest waiting time between when a patient visits their primary care giver and when they first meet a mental health service provider (Pawlowski and Kiejna 2004). It is not overly surprising then, given these facts, that the notion of a quick and relatively easy treatment through a pill may seem an attractive option.

In comparison with other sites, there were noticeably more reservations about pharmacogenomics in Germany. Although many German participants were supportive of pharmacogenomics in a general sense, this support was not without considerable qualification or concern, as detailed in our findings below. It is worthwhile to note here that Germany has some of the lowest prescription rates for antidepressants in the EU and, until recently, it was possible under German social insurance schemes to spend up to one month in a spa, receiving treatment for nerve and psychiatric-related disorders (Rose 2005, Shorter 2005). In this context, it is not hard to see why there may be some reluctance to embrace a genetic test for antidepressants.

In all the groups, choice was a frequently discussed issue – but it was noticeably more so in the English groups, a finding that we attribute to recent initiatives in the NHS promoting patient choice. In all the sites, service users drew heavily on their personal experience of what taking antidepressants meant for them, their friends, family, and fellow mental health service users. There was an overwhelming desire to eliminate adverse drug reactions, as the following excerpts show:

I don't think I would have minded if I, when I was, quite just before I was pinned down, and injected, if they'd have just done a quick swab and actually got me something that wouldn't have been so horrific in its side-effects because my metabolism contradicted it or whatever it is that they use, I don't think I would have minded that actually in a way (English User Group 2).

We realise that our members often do not die of psychiatric disease but of other diseases which they got in effect of the prolonged use of psychotropic drugs, for example liver diseases, stroke, heart failure and many others. It is not unusual for a psychiatric patient to die between the age of 30 or 40. They die because their body can no longer stand so many drugs and it gets ruined. So what most patients dream of is that a medication is formulated that will not bring about side effects. And it is really not important whether it will be developed based on a patient's genotype or in another way. What we really want is that we stop dying prematurely because of the medications we have to take (Polish User Group 3).

Apart from the devastating side effects of medications, users' responses also contained a tenor of desperation regarding their desire to escape from the effects of their illness. One participant reported how his bouts with bipolar illness led him to give away £37,000 without knowing where exactly he had given the money. He conveyed a sense of desperation to end the 'dreadful things' that his disease brought on and the terrible effect it had on his loved ones:

But I mean, certainly, if you were looking for volunteers for the clinical trials here, I would be rushing and banging on your door, because I've nothing to lose, because I do not want to continue the way I am, and I certainly don't want the, the impact that my condition has on my family. I don't want that to continue any longer (English User Group 1).

The sense of helplessness which pervades family members of sufferers from mental illness is captured by a man who lost his wife to depression only the week before agreeing to participate in the focus group:

I am sure that if my wife was given such a chance, perhaps she would have a medication chosen properly and she would still be alive and we would be together. I really cannot say more. Please, forgive . . . Now it is too late for anything and we cannot change it. . . . It's been a week only and I cannot compose. If she had been administered better medications, if there were better medications, perhaps she would be alive now (Polish User Group 1).

Our data seem to confirm other studies which claim that the public is optimistic about the prospects of genomic-based medications (Gaskell *et al.* 2006, Nielsen and Moldrup 2007, Rogausch *et al.* 2006, Rothstein and Hornung 2003). We stress the word 'claim' here since, as discussed above, most people had not heard of pharmacogenomics before being asked their views about it. It is not surprising, therefore, that people who are suffering would have favourable views of a technology that offers them a glimmer of relief. One of the more detailed studies into public views was carried out by the British Royal Society who held a series of public workshops with 76 participants (Royal Society 2005a; 2005b). Although only 'one person per group' had previously heard of pharmacogenomics before attending the workshop, in general, participants were supportive of pharmacogenomic testing as a means of learning more about treatment options and diseases affecting them.

Whilst our work echoes this general approval of genome-based treatments, we also found a number of important themes which will possibly cast a shadow on the acceptance and clinical adoption of pharmacogenomics. In our view, it is crucial to note that none of these studies asked about pharmacogenomic medicines for psychiatric illness. The Royal Society, for example, limited itself to heart disease, cancer, diabetes and asthma. Our data find that whilst there are significant levels of support for pharmacogenomic drugs, there are considerable and significant caveats which are bound to impact on public and user acceptability of pharmacogenomic tests for antidepressants. One theme from our work is that there is a clear difference between mental and physical illness, a difference which may impact on the reception of pharmacogenomics. Below, we explore these reservations.

Drug reactions and disease risks

A key distinction in pharmacogenomics is whether the test sample derives from an infected tissue, *i.e.* a tumour genome, or through blood tests, which unlike cancerous tissue, can reveal the inherited genetics of an individual. Tests for Herceptin, for instance, derive from cancerous tissue whilst those for CYP2D6 metabolism (implicated in antidepressant use) require a blood test, which means that secondary information other than drug reaction results could potentially be discovered. This is because the CYP2D6 is also associated in the metabolism of many other different kinds of medicines. In addition, in some cases, the same genes involved in drug metabolism are also associated with increased risk of other disease conditions (Smart, Martin and Parker 2004).

The Royal Society study cited above aimed to distinguish between the likelihood of 'specific public issues related to pharmacogenomic testing and genetic testing in general' (2005b: 3). The study concluded that 'participants were able to understand easily the basic principles of such testing and its distinction from other genetic tests' (2005b: 6). And yet, crucially, the Royal Society dodged the key issue, since the topic of 'multiple gene interactions in relation to drug metabolism was not discussed.' (2005b: 6: fn6) This is important since it is through such interactions that clinically relevant secondary information is likely to emerge (Netzer and Biller-Andorno 2004).

A mainstream view amongst proponents of pharmacogenomics is that there is no real risk of learning clinically relevant information from a pharmacogenomics test (for example, see Roses 2000). A number of sociological studies, however, are increasingly putting this belief in doubt (Pieri and Wynne 2007, Hedgecoe and Martin 2003, Hedgecoe 2004). Our study found that perceptions of the distinction between susceptibility and treatability are tenuous at best. Representatives in our Policy Workshop indicated that 'there's going to be a blur' between disease risk and drug reaction and 'that blur may be quite large'. As one delegate summarised:

I think it's true as to everybody seems to be saying around the table that you know, with some exceptions, it's difficult to separate out questions about treatability from questions about aetiology, from questions about risk. And questions about risk involve questions about inheritance (Policy Workshop).

Whilst focus group participants understood the difference between testing for drug response and testing for disease risk, this separation was nearly impossible to maintain in actual discussions. There was a sense that 'at the end of the day, a genetic test is a diagnostic method that gives information on a person' (German Public Group 3). There was a belief that various pressures would conspire to make it hard to keep testing at the level of treatability and that usages of test information could 'spread like ripples in the water' (Danish Public Group 3).

A good example of the conflation of disease risk and drug reaction can be found in the exchange below:

A: I would want to know that I was getting the best medication. I'd go for a genetic test if he thought I was depressed or is it, yeah, I would want to know. It's in my interest I feel to be treated properly and I wouldn't want to be depressed so you know, that's just the way I feel. I'd want to be treated properly.

B: Another concern is well where all this genetic results get held, do they get held in a mainframe computer somewhere (multiple voices)

A: I couldn't give tuppence, I couldn't give tuppence where they're held, stored my (multiple voices)

B: Or what they used it for?

A: Or what they used it for. If it's going to benefit me and my family in the long run, then I'm all for it. I mean I would hope you know, my granddaughters are going to be tested to show that they've not got the gene that I may well have passed on to them. And if there's any medication they can take when they get to a certain age that would prevent them from probably getting the same disease, I'd be really happy. I'm only sorry that I didn't know about it sooner (English Public Group 2).

This exchange is useful, for it highlights the interactional contextual of how people react to being asked for a pharmacogenomic test. 'A' is forced to defend his support of pharmacogenomics by a participant who raises her concerns about the storage and future use of test results. Whereas he first expressed his desire to have a test to be 'treated properly' (with the hesitation, 'or, is it', which implies he may not have been absolutely certain as to the aim of the test), 'A' then seems to respond to the possibility of these concerns by conflating susceptibility and treatability and by saying that he would want his granddaughters tested to make sure they were not carriers of a gene that would pre-dispose them to his same disease[5]. We highlight this exchange to bring attention to the point that medical treatment is not a two-person exchange system. Pill taking is invariably a social act (Karp 2004) and it is through a network of significant others that a patient will come to question the wisdom of medicating themselves or the effects of a test on their family and friends.

Difficulty, however, in maintaining a clear distinction and concerns over what a test may yield are only one element that may have an impact on the uptake of pharmacogenomic tests for depression. At the heart of the issue for many is the nature of the illness itself and beliefs about its cause and treatability.

The medical model of depression and antidepressants

Kramer (2005) writes tellingly:

> The anatomical account of depression has changed the way doctors view their patients. The depressed person sits before us. She speaks, wretchedly, of the trivial disappointment that threw her life into a living hell. Hearing of vulnerability in daily life, we imagine vulnerability at the level of the neuron. No need to look to the face and habit. We can imagine glial cells retreating, and neurons withering, at this very moment (2005: 61–2).

The biomedical explanation of depression and antidepressant medication, which Kramer so colourfully embraces, implies that a chemical deficiency in the brain can be treated with drugs which raise the level of amines and alleviates the depression. Perhaps, as Karp argues, the 'necessary condition for widespread psychiatric drug use is a cultural induced readiness to view emotional pain as a disease requiring medical intervention' (Karp 2004: 15). But as an increasing number of commentators are arguing, it does not follow that if enhancing the transmission of serotonin improves depression, then a deficiency in the serotonin system is necessarily responsible for the emergence of the condition in the first place (Horwitz and Wakefield 2007).

For all the support in our focus groups for pharmacogenomics, criticism of the medical model was reflected in a number of responses. There was a feeling that pharmacogenomics represented an extension of the medical model that already pervades the diagnosis and treatment of depression and that 'there might be a bigger incentive to use medicine instead of conversation therapy' if genome-based therapies reached the clinic (Danish Public Group 1). As one member put it:

But the question is whether one should not invest all this money that is used to develop these tests and drugs in other things, like . . . I don't know . . . like social structures that would make people less sick in the first place . . . What is important is that more people start thinking more about these themes and that they maybe have the idea that it is maybe not necessarily the solution to find more efficient drugs. Rather [the solution is to] try to live in another more human society so that one gets less sick and less depressive in the first place (German Public Group 3).

Some service users in the ENUSP organisation (European Network of (ex) Users and Survivors of Psychiatry) explicitly used the term 'the medical model' thus tying their discussion into user/survivor politics:

If I got this questionnaire, going back a couple of months ago, when I was quite unwell, I would have jumped at the chance of a blood test to make me better. But when I would be getting a bit better and I'd start thinking about it more logically, I'd realise that I'm going back into the medical model again and I'm going back into all this, you know, taking drugs (ENUSP).

This quote highlights a related theme that a number of people expressed – that is, a continual fluctuation and/or contradiction in attitude towards their condition and medication. For some users at least, desperation gets entangled with hesitation, depending where/when in the process they are confronted about the possibility of pharmacogenomics.

Ambivalence

In a recent study, Grime and Pollock (2002) interviewed 32 primary care patients diagnosed with mild to moderate depression in the UK and found that many patients held 'shifting perspectives' towards their medication and were full of doubt, ambivalence and uncertainty (2002: 517). On the one hand, people wanted to continue taking antidepressants if it kept their symptoms away and yet simultaneously felt that they were 'weaker' for needing to stay on the drugs and desired to 'sort themselves out' without recourse to medicine. As a result, patients self-adjusted their dosages and concealed this fact from their physician. Feelings of ambivalence were also heightened by the fact that patients could not fathom staying on antidepressants indefinitely, even when they were effective.

Feelings of doubt, uncertainty and ambivalence can also be seen in both public and users' views – not only towards antidepressants but towards depression itself, and towards genetic research. Of course, to some extent this is not surprising since ethical issues surrounding genetics and debates over therapeutic enhancement are well rehearsed. But it seems worth reflecting on this issue since shifting views towards medication targeted for pharmacogenomics research and ambivalence regarding the condition those medicines are designed to treat may well have an impact on the reception of pharmacogenomics tests in the clinic. This is a factor that clinicians, psychiatrists, and health care providers will find hard to ignore when consenting for and prescribing genome-based tests for antidepressants and then monitoring patients' use afterwards.

As one participant put it:

I have friends and colleagues who are taking antidepressants, and I think it has very different effects on them, there are some of them where I can't tell the difference, but some of them have completely lost their personality, and some where it has helped them in a positive way, some of those who have lost their personality, you cannot 'talk' to them any more, I think that is really sad (Danish Public Group 1).

Another indicated that:

> I am actually quite morally ambivalent, because I can see that the individual needs it when that person gets out there, there is really a need for it, when you are completely desperate, when you look at a person with this illness etc. But generally speaking – when you look at it from above – then I think it is dangerous (Danish Public Group 2).

Part of the ambivalence we are aiming to describe relates to depression itself. There was a sense amongst many that depression was 'subjective', that it was not always in need of immediate cure and could in fact be a source of personal growth:

> I think behind [genetic research] is such a conception of human being and also of the illness – now you will be fixed, all will be all right. And I have to say my psychosis was also somehow a process of insight. It was also an experience and I know, not everyone thinks that way but I have undergone it and I didn't want to be repaired at all costs (German User Group).

> It is ambivalence. Only in the cases of small communities is it a sympathetic ambivalence, a positive one. We don't get in your way, you don't get in ours, but okay. You are a member of our community. Whatever happens, we'll stick together. In a city, people are concerned with their own matters, they don't want to think about, engage or look after people who are 'relatively abnormal' (Polish Public Group 1).

Many of our results confirm research done by Karp (1996, 2004). His work, based on one-to-one interviews with users of antidepressants, raised several key themes. First, the decision to go on an antidepressant was rarely taken lightly and was often connected to others' views of the mental condition itself. Secondly, people sought to give meaning to and impose order on their illness and medication use, and these meanings shifted over time. Thirdly, Karp also found that there was a reluctance to see oneself as mentally ill or as needing medication. People reported a general uneasiness about controlling one's feelings with a pill, as against wanting to 'tough it out' (2004: 104).

One can easily surmise that having to undergo a pharmacogenomic test may add another layer of ambivalence to this equation. If patients associate feelings of self-esteem and integrity with their ability to handle personal problems, then what impact will this have on the uptake of the pharmacogenomics of antidepressants?

Depression is not like cancer

A final related theme which emerged from both the public and user groups concerns the difference between psychiatric and physical illness. Whilst the distinction between the two is debatable in medical terms, in social terms the divide is clear. There is an assumption that the symptoms of mental disorders are in some sense less 'real' than those of physical disorders which have a tangible local pathology (Kendell 2001). One group explicitly tied views of depression to those of cancer:

> A: If someone goes to an oncologist, people feel sorry for them.
> B: Exactly, there isn't, in Polish society such a . . . with the other afflictions, that you sympathise, you say 'it's a shame that you are ill'. And yet with psychological problems, then you don't feel sorry for them, you just reject the person (Polish Public Group 3).

Another drew similar conclusions that somehow physical ailments were more 'real':

> Just think for people it's difficult to come to terms with it because if you've got a lump
> or a pain, it's very real. You can go to a doctor and you can show them the lump and
> you can tell them where the pain is. But we're talking about something that's in
> somebody's head and I think that has all kinds of kind of taboos in it
> (English Public Group 1).

And underlying these discussions, of course, is the pervasiveness of stigma that is associated with mental illness:

> A: I think it is much worse to be mentally ill than being physically ill, because you
>   become another person. It is more difficult to feel compassion and people become
>   tired of you
> B: That is exactly it
> A: Your surroundings have a hard time relating to it
> C: And the mentally ill can be a pain in the ass sometimes, phew
> A: And it is hard to know what is right to do, should you pad them, or should you say
>   stop it, damn it (Danish Public Group 2).

Conclusion

In his case study of Herceptin and Tacrine, Hedgecoe (2004) argues that:

> The role of the clinical context is key in shaping the final form of a pharmacogenetic
> technology, and since clinical context is in turn formed by social, cultural and, most of
> all, economic factors, it is these that we should pay attention to when considering the
> broader aspects of personalised medicine (2004: 175).

Whilst pharmacogenomics has broad support, several strong social and cultural themes have emerged from our study, which lead us to argue that discussions of the clinical acceptability of genome-based therapies for depression cannot ignore some of the wider issues regarding depression and antidepressants. These themes include:

1. a tendency to conflate the notions of a pharmacogenomic test for antidepressants with
   a genetic test for depression, a conflation which could cause patients to refuse a
   pharmacogenomic test if they thought (rightly or not) that the results would have wider
   implications for themselves or their relatives.
2. doubts about the medical model of depression, a model which in the minds of some
   people at least does not adequately explain life events as causal factors. More
   importantly for the uptake of pharmacogenomics, there is a related view that the treatment
   of depression has been overly medicalised, leading to a neglect of alterative therapies
   which could be just as efficacious.
       It is worth lingering on this point since, in the UK, the Mental Health Foundation
   has recently advocated that GPs prescribe exercise for mild to moderate depression
   and not antidepressants. Similarly, the National Institute for Health and Clinical
   Excellence (NICE) issued a set of guidelines for treating depression that recommended
   in cases of mild depression, cognitive behavioural therapy ought to be favoured over

antidepressants since the benefit-risk ratio for drugs was poor (NICE 2003). However, it remains to be seen how these recommendations are to be implemented given the lack of qualified therapists and that, according to one study, English GPs are more influenced by the promotion efforts of drug companies than independent sources (Dobson 2003).

3. a deep ambivalence regarding the use of anti-depressants. On the one hand, there is a strong hope, sometimes borne out of desperation as our data show, that new drugs will alleviate patient suffering. Pharmacogenomics may well be seen as part of what Novas (2006) calls a political economy of hope – where science, activism, and capital come together to promote expectations of success in biomedicine. Yet alongside these hopes for a cure, anti-depressant users consistently report that the decision to start taking the drug is not taken lightly, that they feel a sense of 'giving in' by having to swallow a pill each day to help manage their mood. Users also report, as our data showed, that anti-depressants sometimes affected one's personality so severely that they began to question if they were really 'themselves' anymore. Again, the pharmacogenomics of depression cannot separate itself from these issues or from the political and economic context in which the drugs and genetic tests are developed and promoted. It is likely that the ambivalence captured in our groups is re-enforced by media coverage of claims of withheld evidence from clinical trials, antidepressant-induced suicide and murder, class-action law suits, and parliamentary investigations into their power and influence – all of which have recently tarnished the reputation of Eli Lilly and Glaxo Smith Kline (House of Commons 2005).

4. a belief that psychiatric illness is different from physical illness and that depression carries with it a certain cultural value. It is well known that many believe there is a connection between melancholy and artistic talent. As we have seen, some patients consider depression to be 'part of themselves', which they are not sure they would want to lose – despite its considerable stigma. This seems to be very different from the way people talk about having diabetes, heart disease or cancer – a difference, we argue, that may well carry implications for the uptake of pharmacogenomic tests.

Based on data presented here, there exists an ambivalence regarding the personal and cultural significance accorded to depression and anti-depressants (not to mention genetic technology, of course). It is our view that requiring a genetic test in order to be given an anti-depressant adds another reason to question what is already, for some, a life-changing decision, another reason to doubt the medical model of disease causation, and another reason to ask if they are better off living with their depression than treating it with a pill.

Our findings suggest several implications for emerging medical technologies. It seems likely that how, where, and when a technology is adopted will depend, in part, on more than its clinical utility. Social attitudes towards the condition that a technology aims to treat, as well as beliefs about alternative therapies and their perceived efficacy may also influence their introduction into the clinic. Just as important, it is worth noting that patients can hold inconsistent views on these issues. As we have seen, they may place great hope on the prospect of a successful technology, and yet simultaneously may be wary of the assumptions and scientific models underpinning the development of the same technology. In our view, this means that advocates of a new therapy cannot assume that because it promises to work better, it will necessarily be greeted with widespread enthusiasm.

The sociology of expectations reminds us that the future of a technology is co-constructed (Hedgecoe and Martin 2003). In the case of the pharmacogenomics of depression, then, it will not only be the pharmaceutical companies, scientists, and policy makers that shape the field's development. As we have seen, Prozac is not Herceptin and depression is not cancer. Amongst the public and amongst mental health service users, there exists a widespread uncertainty about the nature, cause and meaning of depression as well as a critical reservation about drugs that have moods as their target. The message seems clear: the development and reception of pharmacogenomics of depression will not be reduced to mere efficacy and adverse drug reactions.

Notes

1 We by no means attribute the rise in antidepressant use merely to higher rates of depression. Antidepressants are commonly prescribed for other conditions such as panic attacks, social phobias, and obsessive-compulsive disorders. Again, we highlight this topic at the end of the chapter.
2 Options include the design of new drugs aimed at persons with particular genetic sub-types, the 'rescue' of drugs that have been researched but never made it to market because clinical trial failure, the refinement of drugs already on trial to target particular genetic groups, or tests to screen patients prior to prescription.
3 We are aware that the term 'public' is problematic and we use it here only to distinguish non mental health service users.
4 As explored in the chapter, data show that whilst these groups held strong opinions against pharmacogenomics, some of the themes they raised also emerged in our public groups and with other user organisations.
5 We set aside the fact, of course, that such a test is at present an impossibility for depression and that family history would be a far better indicator anyway.

References

Brown, N. (2003) Hope against hype: accountability in biopasts, presents and futures, *Science Studies*, 16, 3–21.
Clark, C.C., Scott E.A., Boydell, K.M. and Goering, P. (1999) Effects of client interviewers on client reported satisfaction with mental health services, *Psychiatric Services*, 50, 961–3.
Dobson, R. (2003) Pharmaceutical industry is main influence in GP prescribing, *British Medical Journal*, 326, 301.
Gaskell, G., Allansdottir, A., Allum, N., *et al.* (2006) Europeans and biotechnology in 2005: patterns and trends., *Eurobarometer*, 64, 3, Brussels.
Grime, J. and Pollock, K. (2003) Patients' ambivalence about taking antidepressants: a qualitative study, *The Pharmaceutical Journal*, 271, 516–18.
Hedgecoe, A. (2004) *The Politics of Personalised Medicine: Pharmacogenetics in the Clinic*. Cambridge: Cambridge University Press.
Hedgecoe, A. and Martin, P. (2003) The drugs don't work: expectations and the shaping of pharmacogenetics, *Social Studies of Science*, 33, 327–64.
Horwitz, A. and Wakefield, J. (2007) *The Loss of Sadness: how Psychiatry Transformed Normal Sorrow into Depressive Disorder*. Oxford: Oxford University Press.
House of Commons (2005) *The Influence of the Pharmaceutical Industry*. Health Committee Fourth Report of Session 2004–2005 Volume I. London: The Stationery Office Limited.
Karp, D. (1997) *Speaking of Sadness: Depression, Disconnection, and the Meanings of Illness*. Oxford: Oxford University Press.
Karp, D. (2006) *Is it Me or my Meds? Living with Antidepressants*. Cambridge: Harvard University Press.
Kramer, P. (2005) *Against Depression*. New York: Penguin.
Kendell, R. (2001) The distinction between mental and physical illness, *The British Journal of Psychiatry*, 178, 490–3.

Kitzinger, J. (1994) The methodology of focus groups: the importance of interaction between research participants, *Sociology of Health and Illness*, 16, 1, 103–21.

Lindpaintner, K. (2002) The impact of pharmacogenomics and pharmacogenomics on drug discovery, *Nature Reviews*, 1, 463–9.

Martin, P., Lewis, G., Smart, A. and Webster, A. (2006) *False Positive? The Commercial and Clinical Development of Pharmacogenetics.* IGBis, SATSU, University of Nottingham.

Medicines and Healthcare Products Regulatory Agency (2004) Selective serotonin reuptake inhibitor (SSRI) antidepressants – findings of the Committee on Safety of Medicines (CSM) Working Group. Annex A – prescribing trends for SSRIs and related antidepressants. London: MHRA.

National Institute of Clinical Excellence (2003) *Depression: Management of Depression in Primary and Secondary Care, Clinical Guideline 23.* London: National Institute of Clinical Excellence.

Netzer, C. and Biller-Andorno, N. (2004) Pharmacogenomic testing: informed consent and the problem of secondary information, *Bioethics*, 18, 344–60.

Nielsen, L.F. and Moldrup, C. (2007) The diffusion of innovation: factors influencing the uptake of pharmacogenetics, *Community Genetics*, 10, 231–41.

Novas, C. (2006) The political economy of hope: patients' organisations, science, and biovalue, *Biosocieties*, 1, 289–305.

Pawlowski, T. and Kiejna, A. (2004) Pathways to psychiatric care and reform of the public health care system in Poland, *European Psychiatry*, 19, 168–71.

Pieri, E. and Wynne, B. (2007) A qualitative study of personalised medicine: public priorities and values. 'Genetics and Society: Retrospects and Prospects'. CESAGen/CSG 4th International Conference, 26th–28th March 2007, The Royal Society, London.

Rogausch, A., Prause, D., Schallenberg, A., Brockmöller, J. and Himmel, W. (2006) Patients' and physicians' perspectives on pharmacogenetic testing, *Pharmacogenomics*, 7, 49–59.

Rose, D., Wykes, T., Leese, M., Bindman, J. and Fleischmann, P. (2003) Patients' perspectives on electroconvulsive therapy: systematic review, *British Medical Journal*, 326, 1363–6.

Rose, N. (2005) Psycho-pharmaceuticals in Europe. In Knapp, M., McDaid, D., Mossialos, E. and Thornicroft, G. (eds) *Mental Health Policy and Practice across Europe.* Maidenhead: Open University Press.

Roses, A.D. (2000) Pharmacogenomics and the practice of medicine, *Nature*, 405, 857–65.

Rothstein, M.A. and Hornung, C.A. (2003) Public attitudes about pharmacogenomics. In Rothstein, M.A. (ed.) *Pharmacogenomics: Social, Ethical, and Clinical Dimensions.* Hoboken, NJ: John Wiley and Sons.

Royal Society (2005a) *Personalised Medicines: Hopes and Realities.* London: Royal Society.

Royal Society (2005b) *Pharmacogenetics: Dialogue.* London: Royal Society.

Shorter, E. (2005) The historical development of mental health services in Europe. In Knapp, M., McDaid, D., Mossialos, E. and Thornicroft, G. (eds) *Mental Health Policy and Practice across Europe.* Maidenhead: Open University Press.

Silverman, D. (2000) *Doing Qualitative Research.* London: SAGE.

Smart, A., Martin, P. and Parker, M. (2004) Tailored medicine: whom will it fit? Ethics of patient and disease stratification, *Bioethics*, 18, 322–43.

Solomon, A. (2002) *The Noonday Demon: an Anatomy of Depression.* London: Vintage Books.

Vedantam, S. (2004) Antidepressant use by US adults soars, *Washington Post* 3rd December, A15.

Wilkinson, S. (2005) Analysing interaction in focus groups. In Drew, P., Raymond, G. and Weinberg, D. (eds) *Talking Research.* London: SAGE.

World Health Organization (2001) *World Health Report 2001.* Geneva: World Health Organization.

11

Shifting paradigms? Reflections on regenerative medicine, embryonic stem cells and pharmaceuticals

Steven P. Wainwright, Mike Michael and Clare Williams

Introduction

Human embryonic stem (hES) cells are often viewed as heralding the dawn of a revolutionary new age of curative regenerative medicine (Williams *et al.* 2003, Braude and Minger 2005, Kitzinger and Williams 2005) so that 'it seems that every second [news] item is about embryonic stem cells' (Landecker 2007: 233). Our main goal in this chapter is to discuss scientists' views on the possible emergence of a new paradigm of regenerative medicine, the 'disease in a dish' approach to stem cell translation, where it is argued that hES cells will be used as tools for investigating the mechanisms of disease in order to enable the development of new drugs (Department of Health 2005). This is contrasted with the traditional cell transplant paradigm which largely underpins the huge recent expansion in embryonic stem cell research (Lanza *et al.* 2004). For example, almost all of the three billion dollars that is due to be spent on stem cell research in California over the next decade will fund basic research on the biology of human embryonic stem cells (Dalton 2005).

We draw upon Bourdieu's (*e.g.* 1984) analytic schema in order to trace the emerging 'field' of stem cell research, not least as it relates to the links between 'the bench and the bedside' – so-called translational research (Gearhart 2005). In addition, we also make use of recent developments in science and technology studies (STS), namely the sociology of expectations (Brown and Michael 2003), as a means of unravelling the ways in which scientists construct particular futures in the process of situating themselves within the field of stem cell research. In brief, if Bourdieu can provide a sense of the 'structure' that characterises the field of stem cell research, the sociology of expectations can allow us to show how the future of this structure is performed in order to effect change in the present.

In what follows we briefly introduce the theoretical tools that we can derive from the work of Bourdieu and the sociology of expectations. We then go on to examine how scientists and clinicians argue that Pharma resists stem cell transplant strategies, as their large-scale therapeutic use could potentially undermine the pharmaceutical industry. Many of the experts we interviewed, however, also argued that large-scale translational research requires the involvement of 'Pharma' (we use their term throughout our chapter), and that using hES cell lines to study the genetics of 'diseases in a dish' to develop pharmacological therapies is likely to become increasingly important (Scott 2006). In the UK, for example, scientists have pioneered such uses of hES cells, through the innovative use of Pre-Implantation Genetic Diagnosis (PGD) embryos to create stem cell lines with a genetic disease (Pickering *et al.* 2005), whilst in the US 'disease in a dish' approaches are becoming a major model of stem cell translation (Mooney 2005). In this context, we explore the shifting expectations that underpin the possible 'disease in a dish' paradigm of stem cell translation. We conclude with some reflections on the broader implications of our analytic efforts.

Note on methods

In this chapter we use data from two ESRC-funded projects on the prospects and problems of translational research in the field of stem cell research. We draw on over 60 in-depth interviews with scientists and clinicians in some of the leading labs and clinics in the UK and the USA, exploring their views on the bench-bedside interface in the fields of neuroscience and diabetes. The interviews lasted from one to two hours, took place in the experts' offices, and, with permission, were taped and transcribed. Open-ended questions and an informal interview schedule were used in order to encourage scientists and clinicians to speak in their own words about their experiences. Transcripts were analysed by content for emergent themes (Weber 1990), which were then coded (Strauss 1987). The research team discussed the data and analysis which enabled different perspectives to be incorporated, and which added to the richness of the analysis. The respondents' quotes drawn on below were chosen as representative, and illustrate saturated themes. In terms of our analytic approach to these data, this drew on discourse analysis methods (*e.g.* Potter and Wetherell, 1987) which focus upon what accounts 'do' performatively, as opposed to what they represent. On this score, we are less interested in the 'truth-value' of respondents' accounts, than in their capacity to project futures which can have effects.

Bourdieu, the sociology of expectations and stem cell research

Bourdieu's influential concepts of habitus, field and capital, whilst having had a major impact on anthropology, geography and sociology (*e.g.* Williams 1995, Wainwright, Williams and Turner 2006), have had little influence on STS, though Bourdieu's posthumous book – a plea for the use of his ideas in the field of science studies (Bourdieu 2004) – may change that (see Burri 2008). For our part, we attempt to take up his challenge by adopting and adapting Bourdieu's ideas as a means of theorising the 'structures' of the stem cell research field in which the entwinement of academia and the Pharma industry enable the emergence of disease in a dish approaches to regenerative medicine.

Bourdieu's sociology of culture is essentially an account of social practices that can be represented as follows: Habitus + Capital + Field = Practice (Bourdieu 1984: 101). In brief, a *field* is a structured system of social positions and it is within fields that we attain our *habitus*, an 'acquired system of generative dispositions' (Bourdieu 1977: 95) that gives us 'a feel for the game'. Thus, 'when habitus encounters a social world of which it is the product, it is like a 'fish in water' (Bourdieu and Wacquant 1992: 127). Feeling at home in a particular field also depends on our acquisition of four varieties of *capital*: *economic capital* (money etc), *symbolic capital* (prestige; recognition of economic / cultural capital), *social capital* (relations with 'significant others'), and *cultural capital* (legitimate knowledge). In fields like that of embryonic stem cell research, other forms of capital also need to be displayed, most obviously *ethical capital*. Failure to do this can have major repercussions, as the example of 'Hwang-gate' – the case of the disgraced South Korean 'stem cell cloning pioneer' – vividly illustrates (Gottweiss and Treindl 2006).

In the field of science, Bourdieu's main forms of capital can be brought together as *scientific capital*, an amalgam of economic, symbolic, social and cultural capitals. One example of the usefulness of the concept has been examined in a recent Bourdieusian study of the sociology of medical education in the UK, which was seen as a struggle between clinical capital and scientific capital (Brosnan 2008). One medical school was clinically oriented and more closely linked to the health-care field, whilst another adopted a science-oriented curriculum and sought recognition within higher education, a field where scientific capital is more readily translated into economic, cultural and symbolic capital (through research grant income, papers in prestigious journals, dominant positions in university league tables etc).

A further evocative example of the way in which scientists think of the uneven distribution of such 'scientific capital' is given by an eminent scientist (a Fellow of the Royal Society) who asserted that in UK science: 'there's London, Oxford and Cambridge – and then it's a desert until you reach Edinburgh!' (Scientist 13, UK). Here we see another aspect of a Bourdieusian analytic, namely that fields invariably involve struggles for power which reflect the habitus and capital of particular positions within a field.

These notions of 'ethical capital', 'scientific capital', and 'expectational capital' (see below) are useful, and are worth differentiating from the more standard economic, social, symbolic and cultural forms of capital, insofar as they more directly address the specific field with which we are concerned, namely that of stem cell innovation. That is to say, they are heuristics for illuminating the dynamics of this field, even as they are analytically derived from the specificity of this field. On this score, we elaborate on Bourdieu's analytic by taking a Whiteheadian tack (*e.g.* Halewood and Michael in press) which questions the necessary utility of stabilised – or overly 'concretised' – economic, social, symbolic and cultural forms of capital. Accordingly, by focusing upon the *specificity* of the field (of hESC research) we derive the capitals specific to that field which might be particular combinations of economic, social, symbolic and cultural forms of capital, or might include additional capitals (*e.g.* under the 'object turn' that might include 'nature'; see Latour 2004). In other words, our uses of expectational capital reflect what we interpret to be a key characteristic of the field of hESC research – we make no claims about its generaliseability.

Our use of capital can be clarified further. Arguably, capital is itself only productive through some form of display or enactment. That is to say, 'capital' (in our case, for instance, scientific capital) is 'habitually' (that is, 'resourced' by one's habitus) enacted in relation to a field in which such displays are readily read. The eminence of the scientist quoted above is at once presupposed in his statement, and at the same time enacted and reproduced in the statement. The scientist is 'habitually' enacting and reproducing a pattern of inequalities that, within this field, indexes the performative implication that 'success breeds success' as capital begets more capital. Moreover, his is a statement about the future – it performs the temporal continuity of a world of *élites* distributed in a particular way and, in so doing, 'aspires' to reproduce that world in the present and, indeed, future. In other words, such 'habitual' displays of capital are moves in a game that is fundamentally oriented to the future. Past and present scientific capital are employed to accumulate future scientific capital.

This brief reading of Bourdieu's analytic schema (albeit succinctly presented here) is clearly influenced by the emerging area of sociology of expectations, or at least that perspective in the sociology of expectations that emphasises performativity and places particular focus upon the discursive enactment of future hopes. As such, this variant of the sociology of expectations analyses the 'hope and hype' discourses and practices of scientists (*e.g.* Brown 2003, Wainwright *et al.* 2006a, Michael *et al.* 2007b). As Brown and Michael (2003) have shown, these accounts typically reflect on the prospects for new medical technologies both at the moment of providing the account, and also upon prior expectations about such prospects. In other words, scientists and clinicians are able to place research in the broader context in which past expectations (and their accuracy or otherwise) colour current expectations (Kitzinger and Williams 2005). Such discourses, narratives and accounts are interesting not so much in terms of what they 'represent' (current beliefs, the past etc), but rather in terms of what they 'do' (*e.g.* Gilbert and Mulkay 1984, Potter and Wetherell 1987). Thus, a key focus of the sociology of expectations is in the practices by which such discourses are put into circulation, for example, the material form statements take, the routes of their dissemination, their timing (Hedgecoe 2004).

In this chapter, we will trace how stem cell scientists, in demarcating persuasive futures in the present with a view to making both present and future, enact what we might tentatively call *expectational capital*. By this we mean to suggest that their versions of the future reflect and intervene in a stem cell research field in which they are able to make *only particular 'moves'* – moves that respond to what are perceived as the 'future realities' of the field – future realities that are, as we will see, influenced by the perceived role of Pharma, among others. Needless to say, there are numerous dimensions to expectational capital that we cannot explore in any detail here. For example, we can imagine that such 'moves' are as much about maintaining expectational capital within the field – that is, the ostensible capacity to make credible statements about future events. Further, these moves are not simply social, but are partially connected to the heterogeneous relations that make up the 'natures' of embryonic stem cells (Michael *et al.* 2007a, 2007b).

This last point brings us to a further consideration of another peculiarity of our analytic perspective. We are aware that other work in the sociology of expectations literature highlights the mediation of expectations in heterogeneous relations that can take such forms, artefacts, technologies, scientific fields, institutions, regulatory regimes, etc (see, for instance, van Lente 1993, Hedgecoe and Martin 2003), some of which can be understood as, or related to, 'structural' concepts (*e.g.* niches, socio-technical systems). These approaches articulate with work on expectations which is more discursive in character (*e.g.* Brown and Michael 2003). However, this articulation has not been *systematically* treated. In response to the question 'To what does Bourdieu's perspective on (structuring) structure add?', we would argue that Bourdieu's concepts of habitus, capital and field provide a *systematic* approach enabling researchers to analyse the ways in which individuals and institutions, but also discourses (or enactments) and 'systems' (or fields) co-produce each other through a 'processing of structure'. Thus, capital confers power and influence within a field and it is through promoting the value of forms of capital at stake in a field that this capital attains value. In our case study, as we hope to show, those who promote the disease in a dish approach are using various forms of capital to add value to their expectational capital, that is, their capacity persuasively to pronounce upon the future. To put this another way, Bourdieu brings to the table an analytic and systematic sensibility that such heterogeneous embodiments of expectations have at some point to be enacted (not least in an emergent and fluid field like stem cell research). Such enactments need to be appropriate to – or 'at home' in – the specific field which will encapsulate disparate and agonistic actors, and which structures how antagonisms can be played out. This neatly resonates with another key concern within the sociology of expectations, namely the focus on 'contested futures' (Brown *et al.* 2000).

In the next two empirical sections, we will present a range of scientists' accounts about the changing field of stem cell research. In particular, in a field in which a key player is Pharma, we trace how particular stem cell futures are respectively truncated and opened up in particular ways.

Stem cells: transplantation versus Pharma?

Several influential science studies texts have argued that there has been a shift from 'pure science' – where the Citadel of Science spoke 'truth to power' – to a model where science has been co-opted into policy and politics, and where science promises to become the productive engine of a new knowledge (bio) economy (*e.g.* Nowotny *et al.* 2001). As Rabinow (1996a) puts it:

> More than ever before, the legitimacy of the life sciences now rests on claims to produce health . . . The bioscience community now runs the risk that merely producing truth

will be insufficient to move the venture capitalists, patent offices, and science writers on whom the biosciences are increasingly dependent for their new found wealth (1996a: 137).

In Bourdieu's terms the fields of science and business have become increasingly interdependent. The assumption behind Rabinow's claim is that scientific breakthroughs should be translated from lab to clinic to market. In the stem cell field these prospective transitions are the reason for the large amount of funding currently going into basic research (around £100 million in the UK). However, in the field of stem cells for diabetes, for instance, progress has been much slower than anticipated:

> I think people were expecting to get to the clinic much faster. Now people are saying, 'Hey, that's not the issue right now, let's see what we need to do to get it so that the *field* moves on' (Scientist 25, USA).

On one level, the reason for this lack of progress lies in the sheer difficulty of making *functioning* cells in the lab over the last five years or so. We have explored elsewhere some of the complex reasons for this lack of progress in the prospective move from the lab to the clinic. As scientists are all too aware, this difficulty is intertwined with various institutional and ethical influences (Wainwright *et al.* 2006a, 2006b, 2007, Michael *et al.* 2007a).

However, this lack of progress is of course constructed and enacted, It conveys a sense of disappointed expectations – expectations that have arisen in a field partly shaped by such factors as governmental funding programmes. Consider the following quote:

> There's millions of pounds of Government money for stem cell research and scientists want this money . . . But I think people are rushing ahead and publishing prematurely. A lot of papers show that the cells look like this, but there's no real proof of real function. Are they any use, do they live, do they differentiate, do they respond to the right physical and environmental cues? (Scientist 40, UK).

This scientist, in criticising the premature rush to publish, can be seen to be reacting to the influx of research money that raises the stakes for scientists who need to maintain their scientific and expectational capital. They must be seen to realise the expectations of the field through publication. Such expectations can also be situated more broadly within changes in contemporary Western temporality characterised by the rise of an 'extended present' in which there is a 'mounting pressure that solutions to impending, recognizable problems have to be found now' (Nowotny 1994: 52).

This problem of 'premature publication', however, is also seen by stem cell scientists as so problematic that even 'stem cell breakthrough papers' which appear in top journals such as *Nature* are routinely treated as just 'too good to be true'. For example, in the diabetes field the feeling is that if a lab really could make functioning beta cells which could cure diabetes then they would patent their process, rather than publish their results:

> *How are you going to turn stem cells into beta cells?*

> If we did know how to do it we would patent it [rather than publish] and be millionaires! (Scientist 4, UK).

Basic bioscience in the West is now tied to the idea of 'producing cures' (and is also tied with nationalistic ideas of world scientific leadership and prestige, as well as a source of economic success which in turn leads us back to 'cures'). For example, translational research is now strongly shaping the biomedical research agenda of the Medical Research Council (MRC) in the UK (MRC 2004), and the National Institutes of Health (NIH) in the USA (Zerhouni 2003). Accordingly, Colin Blakemore, the Director of the MRC, recently stated that:

> Over the coming years we intend to accelerate the rate at which MRC research is translated into new methods of diagnosis and treatment – a process that can take anything from a few years to decades . . . to bring our knowledge and discoveries into the healthcare system and so to patients (MRC 2004: 1).

This is no doubt a laudable aim. However, delivering such translational research from hES cells in the UK is likely to be a difficult task for funding bodies such as the MRC, as a UK scientist explains:

> There's a problem with the pressure that's been put on the MRC in the direction of more and more translational research. They don't have the money for the translation studies! Clinical trials would just be astronomical . . . The MRC and the Wellcome [Trust] should underpin *basic research* studies to a point when they need to become translational, then other organisations should come in . . . This is long-term stuff . . . I asked [a highly placed scientist within MRC] about the money going into stem cells – 'Do you have a list of objectives that you expect to get out of this money in five years' time?' And I don't think there was an answer . . . You would hope that the MRC would have a list of objectives. 'This is the money that's going in, and in five years' time, this is what we'd like to see.' I hope what they haven't got down is 'We want to see this in the clinic in five years,' because I don't think it's going to happen (Scientist 19, UK).

As noted above, there are other difficulties that interdigitate with the sheer scientific difficulty of hES cell research (*e.g.* Wainwright *et al.* 2006a, 2007). Even if ES cells can be made that are suitable for transplantation, this 'proof of principle' research still needs translating into routine therapies. Such routinisation is of course a standard trajectory within biomedicine (*e.g.* PCR – Rabinow 1996b, Cyclosporin – Fox and Swazey 1992). However, it is also a process that is fraught, not least because actors within the field enact expectations about where, and by whom, such expectations about translation should be realised. Echoing the comments of the scientist above, is the UK Department of Health's (2005) *'Pattison Report'* on the development of stem cell research, which claims that translational research is currently a major problem for the stem cell field in the UK. Pattison argues that the role of the MRC etc has been to support basic biomedical research and that historically Pharma has largely funded the move to the clinic. At the launch of his report Sir John Pattison used the metaphor of a translational research 'valley of death' (Highfield 2005) to highlight the need for governments to invest tens of millions of pounds per year in funding translational research (see Moran 2007).

Our interview data, however, suggest that hES cells as potential transplant therapies are not a priority for Pharma, for two main reasons. First, Pharma companies have considerable expertise in bringing small molecule drugs (chemicals) to the clinic, but they currently have little interest in or knowledge of large molecules (proteins, antibodies etc). Secondly, Pharma is particularly reluctant to become involved in something as contested as hES cells (Wainwright *et al.* 2006a), as this could have a significant downward effect on their share price – especially in the huge US market:

> The Pharma companies are not strongly in favour of embryonics . . . They need blockbuster drugs and they think they can use embryonics to discover novel new simple molecules which they can sell by the ton load (Scientist 21, UK).

> The big Pharmas have been exceptionally cagey about the stem cell field for a variety of reasons – one, protecting their current portfolio, and two, you don't want to get into this field and see it go belly up. They're interested in shortcutting the time for drug development (Scientist/Clinician 43, UK).

Pharma also recognises, however, that effective cell therapies could have a huge effect on their market share in diseases such as diabetes:

> If you can turn cells into beta cells and transplant them, there are an awful lot of drug companies that would be very unhappy with that (Scientist 3, UK).

Of course, 'the diabetes industry' includes much more than Pharma companies producing drugs and insulin. For instance, there is also a whole biotech sector that manufactures glucose monitors, sophisticated insulin pump systems and so on. Even here, the contested nature of 'fields within diabetes' is clear. For example, several diabetes cell biologists we interviewed argued for an immunological approach to curing diabetes (despite not being immunologists themselves) which, if successful, would both undermine the scientific field of attempting to create cell transplant treatments for diabetes using stem cells, and also undercut much of the existing 'diabetes industry':

> The 'diabetes industry' is where all the money has been invested. If cell therapy becomes 100 per cent effective we can get rid of *all* the existing therapies. As a matter of fact, I think we are going to prevent diabetes before we can cure it by cell replacement . . . I believe Type-1 diabetes will be prevented through the identification of the antigen, and through vaccines (Scientist/Clinician 49, USA).

The fields of diabetes, stem cells, transplantation and immunology overlap and scientists wedded to a 'cell transplant' approach may have their habitus disrupted by their scientific colleagues in the field of immunology if this group can produce a vaccine as a cure for diabetes. Persuading fellow scientists of the veracity of a particular approach is, of course, only a first step. As we saw earlier, Pharma has a vested interest in maintaining the current 'drug-based' approaches to diabetes.

Let us attempt to summarise this complicated array of accounts. From the perspective of stem cell scientists, the field of stem cell research is characterised by a range of expectations. For organisations such as the MRC, there is an expectation of rapid translation from the laboratory to the clinic; for some scientists and institutions such as the Department of Health, this is problematic not least in terms of how such expectations are to be realised. For other scientists the expectation is still that Pharma is negatively predisposed toward stem cell therapeutics. In terms of expectational capital and its 'habitual' enactment, this (albeit simplified) tripartite configuration of expectations suggests the following:

- The Medical Research Council is situating itself as a player that can oversee the realisation of the expectation of the bench-to-bedside translation. Its expectational capital resides in its capacity to fund such translational research but such capital is likely to be maintained only with the realisation of those expectations;

- The Department of Health's expectations (as articulated in the Pattison report) attempt to undermine the expectational capital of the MRC by setting out a different set of expectations in which the MRC is largely a funder of basic research rather than translation, and other organisations including Pharma can supply their expertise in developing therapies from experimental findings;
- Some scientists dispute this version of the field by suggesting that it is misguided to expect Pharma, which has traditionally played a major translational role, to act in a similar way in relation to stem cell therapeutics. Expectational capital is here enacted in a reorientation to different sorts of futures (*e.g.* immunology).

The last of these actually implies a shift toward the expectations of Pharma, including the production of vaccines. However, as we shall see in the next section, stem cell research too can be re-oriented towards Pharma's expectational capital.

'Disease in a dish': a new paradigm of stem cell research?

In the preceding section, we explored a field characterised by varying expectations about the viability (technical and institutional) of the differentiating stem cells into functioning cells. In this next section, we turn to a rather different range of expectations that assume that the whole cell transplant approach to translating stem cell into therapies is highly problematic, indeed, wrongheaded. Instead, or at least as well as, many of the scientists we spoke to argued that stem cells should be used as *tools* to study potential new drug therapies rather than as cell *therapies* in their own right. The whole rationale for such a radical shift is captured in a quote from a US scientist:

> Stem cells have been, over the last two or three years, almost explicitly sold to the public as potential therapeutic applications for transplantation, and it is the simplest way to think about it . . . But, people are now asking when are we first going to see the real cure? When are the benefits going to be in the clinic? Is it going to be diabetes? Is it going to Parkinson's Disease? And I think some opportunists have jumped into this field, done some rat studies with human ES cells and some changes occurred. I think that people were shaken and some scientists started backing off and saying it's all hype. There are no real cures in this domain . . . For the last year or so I've been talking about how you can study diseases in a dish through cell culture. This is a revolution in human biology. This is a paradigm shift . . . This is going to happen. It's too clear. It's too right (Scientist 29, USA).

Here we see an almost messianic vision of expectations for revolutionary stem cell biology where diseases in a dish change the face of modern bioscience. The prophecy is that stem cell lines of a disease such as Amyotrophic Lateral Sclerosis (ALS, sometimes called Motor Neurone Disease – MND) will be used to develop new therapies:

> I see disease in a dish stem cell lines as research tools, not clinical tools. They will reveal drugs that might be then used in the clinic – and they will reveal mechanisms that suggest drugs that should be used that may not have been thought about before (Scientist/ Clinician 30, USA).

Proponents of this new approach suggest that there are at least three major ways of producing these disease in a dish stem cell lines. First, it is possible, in principle, to use somatic cell nuclear transfer (SCNT), sometimes called CNR – cell nuclear replacement – and often referred to as 'therapeutic cloning'. Here, an affected cell nucleus, taken from, for example, a skin cell of someone with ALS, is placed into an embryo that has had its nucleus removed (hence CNR). In principle it is then possible to make an hES cell line from this 'affected embryo' and this line would carry the 'genetic mutations' for ALS. All of this looks compelling on an animated Power-point slide – as we have witnessed at many seminars and conferences on stem cells. However, the only paper that claimed to have created 'disease hES cell lines' using this approach is by Professor Hwang's group in South Korea. In this case the paper was retracted when it was subsequently demonstrated that the results were fraudulent. Scientist 29 (above) was speaking to us before 'Hwang-gate' when he suggested that 'disease in a dish' hES cell lines could be produced by CNR. Perhaps they will be, but at this point it may, from a perspective outside biomedical science, seem prudent to rein back expectations on this particular strategy for disease in a dish as the saviour of the hES cell field. Or to put it another way, the Hwang incident has impacted on the expectational capital of all those operating within the field, and expectations must be much more circumspect. That said, the strategy of SCNT remains a high-profile area within the embryonic stem cell field, particularly in the UK where the HFEA has recently allowed the payment of IVF patients (in the form of subsidised treatment) for eggs (in late 2007) and also the derivation of inter-species embryos (*e.g.* using cow eggs and human cells to create disease in a dish ESC lines, in early 2008) on the basis that this is an important potential path to cures.

We emphasise that using somatic cell nuclear transfer in hESC research is pioneering 'science in the making'. A US scientist we interviewed argues that the whole point of doing 'cutting-edge science' is to focus on difficult problems where the prospects of success may be small, but where the rewards are huge:

> With enabling technologies like hESC there will be fundamental shifts in the way problems in human biology and human medicine are tackled . . . If you had a human brain cell with a specific condition like ALS it gives you a way to test drugs, to make drugs, to make therapies. This is good stuff . . . There will be lots of surprises and we wouldn't be scientists if we didn't believe that the happy surprises were going to outweigh the unhappy surprises . . . One idea is that if I take one of your skin cells, and I make an embryonic stem cell line from it . . .

> *But the Hwang paper is now discredited, so no one has done this, so isn't that a problem?*

> I've never been put off by a problem. The important problems are sometimes difficult. And if you look at the magnitude of neurological diseases like Alzheimer's I'd say it's worth putting some really serious effort into it. You don't discover things if you don't look in places where nobody's looked before (Scientist 51, USA).

Here, expectational capital takes on a different, more general, 'habitual' form – that science is pioneering and difficult, and that 'risk taking' is what should be expected of elite scientific research which promises a surfeit of scientific capital.

A second potential approach to creating disease in a dish hES cell lines is to use the highly successful genetic engineering techniques that enable molecular biologists to create 'animal models' of disease. As one of our UK scientists explained, this may prove more productive than attempts to develop cell transplant therapies in areas of neuroscience like ALS:

The motor neurons are sprayed from the top of the motor cortex right down the spinal cord, they're in the core of the spinal cord, and they're the biggest cells in the body. That doesn't sound like a smart target in terms of cell replacement therapy! I really want to see the disease stopped . . . I'm not really working on cellular therapy . . . We are still tempted to do some simple experiments with hES cells transplanted into our mouse model of disease (ALS). It's one of the few really good mouse models of any neuron genetic condition so we're quite lucky in that respect. But that's not the main thrust of my work. I still think that ALS is going to be tackled from a pharmaceutical point of view and that drug discovery is very important . . . So diseases in a dish, that's exactly the kind of research I do (Scientist/Clinician 33, UK).

Here, pharmaceutical approaches are seen as trumping cell transplant strategies. Expectational capital is enacted primarily in terms of the physiological facts: the extended nature of motor neurons. That is to say, scientific capital that enables pronouncements on the peculiarity of motor neurons is used to negate expectations about stem cell therapeutics. Against this, however, can be posed a number of problems which draw on different sorts of expectational capital. Thus, one problem with this genetic-engineering approach is that you need to know the gene(s) to 'knock-in' to produce a particular disease. Monogenetic diseases, such as Huntingdon's, are good targets for this approach. For other diseases, matters are more complicated. Thus, for ALS, only one gene is known and it is assumed that at least several genes produce ALS – in other words, the 'disease model' of ALS is only a partial representation of ALS. This is not to say that such a model is worthless, but extrapolating from the 'knock-in model' to patients with ALS is fraught with difficulties. In addition, many diseases are polygenetic and this complexity is difficult to wholly produce via traditional genetic-engineering approaches (*e.g.* to produce 'models' of diabetes) – whether these are animal models or 'disease in a dish' models.

In the last few years, however, there has been some research on the use of a third approach to making disease in a dish hES cell lines through using affected PGD embryos (Williams *et al.* 2008):

PGD lines could be very important . . . stem cells for therapy . . . This is a potential source to study genetic conditions. You could actually look through the very early stages where the genes switch on. What actually happens? Can you change it? Could it be a pharmaceutical target? (Scientist/Clinician 16, UK).

There are currently a few hES cell lines that have been created from PGD embryos, for example, affected with a key Cystic Fibrosis (CF) gene (Pickering *et al.* 2005). What is striking here is that a new set of expectations is being generated for what is, essentially, an untried approach. This approach is 'science-in-the-making' rather than 'ready made science', to use a distinction drawn by Latour (1987). The field of disease in a dish stem cell lines – however they are produced – is so new that few scientists are currently exploring questions such as 'What actually happens? Can you change it? Could it be a pharmaceutical target?' The assumption behind these questions is that scientists *will* unravel the genetic mechanisms of disease, that they *will* change these through (say) genetic engineering, and that they *will* design drugs that work on particular 'pharmaceutical targets' within cells. Such a shift from basic bioscience to medical technologies is, however, something that can only be delivered in the (promised) future. Here, emergent expectations revolve around the scientific capital derived from the capacity to 'speak for' PGD cells that seemingly embody the specificity of particular diseases such as CF. However, such specificity can also be seen as un-scientific (hence, comprising scientific capital) insofar as PGD might fail to accommodate broader scientific principles of experimental practice. Thus, the PGD approach is itself seen as flawed by proponents of the genetic-engineering approach to creating disease in a dish hESC lines:

> I think disease lines from PGD are oversold . . . Is it better to take a bunch of hESC lines that come from different unrelated embryos of unknown genetic architecture, with Huntingdon's say, and compare them with each other? Or is it better to take one cell line where you control the genetic background, and introduce into it the mutations that you want to study? Now to scientists, maybe the answer's obvious. The more things you can control, the fewer variables you have floating around the experiment. So that's the problem I have with a lot of these PGD efforts. I'm not saying that people shouldn't do it; of course they should do it . . . But if you ask me, 'Do I think that's actually a robust approach' I'd say you're better off getting good control so if you want to have multiple genetic backgrounds, put the mutations in two different genetic backgrounds and then you study them in a dish. And then you can actually ask: 'Do they behave exactly the same?' Part of what I was brought up to believe as the best way, the robust way, to do experimental science is to set things up so that you're changing one thing at a time, where you can clearly figure out what the contribution is of that one thing, to the best of your ability . . . Just throwing technology at a problem doesn't necessarily give you interpretable data. So I'm very sceptical about how much will come out of these derivations of lines from PGD (Scientist 51, USA).

This view of science as providing rigorous and hence interpretable data is an enactment of scientific capital that waylays the expectations associated with PGD, and opens up the space for expectations associated with genetic engineering. Moreover, the scientist here is also discursively distinguishing between the rigorous science that he performs and 'the other' less scientifically robust approach of those who have more of a clinically oriented background in PGD.

As we might expect, the newer expectations around disease in a dish approaches have themselves been open to criticism. It is easy enough to regard such accounts about the future pharmaceutical prospects of stem cell research as a matter of 'painting targets around arrows'. In other words, the arrow of the expectations of using hES cells for transplant therapies seems to be falling short of the target. By arguing that the arrow of therapies should be the new target of disease in a dish, hES scientists and clinicians can claim that expectations of future treatments are now grounded in what has been accomplished through, for instance, the production of CF hES cell lines from PGD. Alternatively, one can criticise such expectations in terms of their lack of grounding in a rounded knowledge of the disease that extends beyond its reductionist 'manifestation' in the dish:

> Even if we understood everything about stem cells, if you don't know anything about the disease you can't say what you want it to fix. What the lay public, and unfortunately some scientists, and certainly clinicians believe, is that stem cells are like pixie dust. You just sprinkle it on the pathology and magically it will transform things! (Scientist/ Clinician 30, USA).

What is striking here is the way in which this scientist/clinician positions himself positively in relation to 'unethical/unscientific others'.

In summary, we can point to the three expectational positions within the emerging field of disease in a dish: therapeutic cloning, genetic engineering and PGD. Each of these in its own way is expected to generate techniques for studying stem cells that are diseased, with a view to developing pharmaceutical therapies.

This, of course, stands in contrast to the view that stem cells can themselves comprise the therapy. Such a move toward disease in a dish approaches – what we might call the emerging pharmaceutical approach to the field – can be read as a reaction to the yet unfulfilled expectations of stem cell therapy approaches. However, as we saw in the preceding section, 'unfulfilled expectations' arise in fields in which scientific capital is enacted in relation to the expectational capital of research-funding bodies, of governmental bodies and, importantly, of Pharma. That is to say, expectations (and their lack of realisation) are performed in the context of expectations *about* the expectations of particular prominent actors (we have suggested that in the UK these include the MRC, Department of Health, Pharma) who centrally influence the meaning of realisation (or otherwise) of expectations.

In the concluding section, we consider these changing fields of stem cell research in a little more detail, as well as reflecting on our use of Bourdieu's analytic schema in tandem with the sociology of expectations.

Concluding remarks

In this chapter, we have attempted to chart some of the key changes we see in the field of hESC research, especially as performed and projected by actors within that field. We have documented a number of ways in which scientists demarcate the prospects of the field – prospects which address not only the technical dimensions of the science (*e.g.* whether the differentiation of stem cells can be controlled, whether the disease in a dish approach is too reductionist), but also economic, political and social aspects (*e.g.* unrealistic institutional expectations about translation, resistance from Pharma in supporting stem cell therapeutics). In particular, we have explored what we see as the emerging influences of pharmaceuticals in the social shaping of technological options within the emerging embryonic stem cell field. We have explored how this field is being reconfigured in different ways (by the perceived interests of Pharma), and have examined how new stem cell identities are being invented during the process of future making.

These changes have been traced with the aid of Bourdieu's analytic schema in which Bourdieu's standard capitals have been reworked to take into account the specificity of the field of hESC research. Moreover, Bourdieu has also been partially 'read through' the sociology of expectations to derive what we have called scientific and expectational capital. We are acutely aware that the latter perspective's emphasis on the performative has blurred Bourdieu's conceptual distinctions between field, capital and habitus, not least by virtue of our insistence on seeing expectational capital as continuously 'habitually' enacted, and the field continuously characterised and recharacterised. If the sociology of expectations has brought this performative sensibility to Bourdieu, and thus loosened up the more conservative – or socially reproductive – dimensions of habitus, field and capital, Bourdieu has brought a systematising sense of the complex structuring *patterns* of expectations that characterise the field, and their association with the array of particular actors (and their expectational capitals, and thus their particular versions of the future). In sum, Bourdieu has served as both a resource and a topic with which to explore the particularities of the hESC research field. His analytic has illuminated our explorations by providing some tools for the '*systematic*' analysis of the 'performative' and the 'stable' (*e.g.* institutional), but only because, treated as a topic, we have read Bourdieu through *performativity* and with an emphasis upon *specificity*.

We are in no doubt that this 'interfacing' of Bourdieu and the sociology of expectations needs considerable elaboration, and ours has been an inevitably partial analysis of the field of hESC research. For instance, our focus on expectational capital could be further elaborated in relation to other forms of capital in its realisation. This is exemplified by economic capital in the form of the financial backing to push a research programme, or social capital in the form of links with important others such as funders, regulators, patient constituencies and other 'techno-scientific stakeholders'. Our aim here has been primarily to make an initial foray into how these two perspectives might conjointly illuminate the evolving field of hESC research. Our 'expectation' is that its extension to other rapidly changing fields might yield insights that would otherwise be missed.

Of the undoubtedly many limitations to the present exploratory chapter, we specify four areas that seem to us to be worthy of future research. First, we acknowledge that the two visions of cell-based therapy and diseases in a dish we have discussed are not mutually exclusive approaches. Indeed, a standard strategy in bioscience is to develop research tools as a means of generating revenue to fund longer-term work on therapies (*e.g.* in the area of oncogenes, see Fujimura 1987) and we anticipate that stem cell scientists will also adopt this twin-track strategy. This is an empirical dimension of the present field that could usefully be further investigated.

Secondly, though we have addressed Pharma primarily in terms of how it is enacted by our respondents, these enactments also derive from the role of Pharma and pharmaceuticals. As recent studies show, Pharma continues to pursue an aggressive marketing approach to producing profits where there's 'a pill for every ill and an ill for every pill' (Blech 2006: 40). In addition, 'Worldwide, images of well-being and health are increasingly associated with access to pharmaceuticals' (Petryna and Keinman 2006: 1). Stem cell scientists in promoting images of the use of stem cells as vital tools for producing valuable new drugs respond to and advance such pharmaceutical visions. As such, one useful way of extending our research would be through gathering data from within the pharmaceutical industry on their expectations of the embryonic stem cell field. Such research would build upon recent research on Pharma's investment in the haematopoetic stem cell field in the 1990s (see Brown *et al.* 2006).

Thirdly, by highlighting the way in which expectations are enacted, we have laid less stress on the dimension of 'impression management' that is also a pervasive feature of our interview data. By this we mean that our respondents also engage in presenting themselves as particular sorts of actors, not least through forms of identification and differentiation from other actors. For instance, both scientists and clinicians exhibit a 'habitus of othering', differentiating themselves through their expectations of emerging stem cell technologies and thus positioning themselves in relation to the apparent paradigm shift that is taking place. Indeed, at times our informants present themselves less as actors than as acted upon (*e.g.* by such 'others' as the MRC, the DoH, the pharmaceutical industry). This sort of treatment would provide an additional dimension to the analysis presented here.

Finally, it can be argued that our focus upon scientists' enactment of the pharmaceutical shift toward disease in a dish approaches has been rather 'monotone'. To the extent that these scientists' expectations about changes in the field are *clearly* articulated, they are a means to affecting that field in particular ways, but also of *motivating* themselves and their colleagues in a scientific field typically laden with scepticism (see Brown *et al.* 2000). Ironically, such scepticism, as we have hinted above, is part of the scientific capital of scientists, but it can also take various forms that serve in the 'reproduction' of scientific capital. For instance, scepticism toward self – that is, that one might oneself be overly invested in a particular technique (or on board a bandwagon that will only be revealed in the future – see Michael *et al.* 2007a). A second version of scepticism concerns clarity itself: the future cannot be known and to be too clear or definitive about it risks one's scientific capital. As such, vague or ambivalent expectations can themselves be functional within the field (Michael *et al.* 2007b). Taking these points together, and as a means of expanding on the processes of pharmaceutical influences on the embryonic stem cell field, it behoves us to consider in the future how such scepticism and vagueness might be the means by which an emergent perspective on pharmaceutical disease in a dish research and therapies comes to be realised.

References

Blech, J. (2006) *Inventing Disease and Pushing Pills: Pharmaceutical Companies and the Medicalisation of Normal Life*. London: Routledge.
Bourdieu, P. (1977) *Outline of a Theory of Practice*. Cambridge: Cambridge University Press.
Bourdieu, P. (1984) *Distinction: a Social Critique of the Judgement of Taste*. London: Routledge.
Bourdieu, P. (2004) *Science of Science and Reflexivity*. Cambridge: Polity.
Bourdieu, P. and Wacquant, L. (1992) *An Invitation to Reflexive Sociology*. Cambridge: Polity Press.
Braude, P.R. and Minger, S. (2005) Stem cell therapy: hope or hype, *British Medical Journal*, 330, 1159–60.
Brosnan, C.J. (2008) The sociology of medical education: the struggle for legitimate knowledge in two English medical schools. Unpublished PhD Thesis, University of Cambridge.
Brown, N. (2003) Hope against hype: accountability in biopasts, presents and futures, *Science Studies*, 16, 2, 3–21.
Brown, N., Kraft, A. and Martin, P. (2006) The promissory past of blood cells, *BioSocieties*, 1, 329–48.
Brown, N. and Michael, M. (2003) An analysis of changing expectations: or Retrospecting Prospects and Prospecting Retrospects, *Technology Analysis and Strategic Management*, 15, 1, 3–18.
Brown, N., Rappert, B. and Webster, A. (2000) *Contested Futures: a Sociology of Prospective Techno-Science*. Aldershot: Ashgate.
Burri, R.V. (2008) Doing distinctions: boundary work and symbolic capital in radiology, *Social Studies of Science*, 38, 35–62.
Dalton, R. (2005) California prepares to roll out stem-cell funding, *Nature*, 7060, 800–1.
Department of Health (2005) *UK Stem Cell Initiative: [Pattison] Report and Recommendations*. London: HMSO.
Fox, R.C. and Swazey, J.P. (1992) *Spare Parts: Organ Replacement in American Society*. New York: Oxford University Press.
Fujimura, J.H. (1987) Constructing 'do-able' problems in cancer research: articulating alignment, *Social Studies of Science*, 5, 257–93.
Gearhart, J. (2005) *Stem Cells: Nuclear Reprogramming and Therapeutic Applications*. Novartis Foundation Symposium. New York: Wiley.
Gilbert, G.N. and Mulkay, M. (1984) *Opening Pandora's Box: a Sociological Analysis of Scientists' Discourse*. Cambridge: Cambridge University Press.
Gottweiss, H. and Triendl, R. (2006) South Korean policy failure and the Hwang debate, *Nature, Biotechnology*, 24, 141–3.
Halewood, M. and Michael, M. (in press) Being a sociologist and becoming a Whiteheadian: concrescing methodological tactics, *Theory, Culture and Society*.
Hedgecoe, A. (2004) *The Politics of Personalised Medicine: Pharmacogenetics in the Clinic*. Cambridge: Cambridge University Press.
Hedgecoe, A. and Martin, P. (2003) The drugs don't work: expectations and the shaping of pharmacogenetics, *Social Studies of Science*, 33, 327–64.

Highfield, R. (2005) Pledge to make Britain 'leading location for research into drugs and treatments'. *Daily Telegraph*, 6th December.

Kitzinger, J. and Williams, C. (2005) Envisaging the future: legitimising hope and calming fears in the stem cell debate, *Social Science and Medicine*, 61, 731–40.

Landecker, H. (2007) *Culturing Life: How Cells Became Technologies*. Cambridge: Harvard University Press.

Lanza, R., Blan, H., Melton, D., *et al*. (2004) *Handbook of Stem Cells, Volume 1 – Embryonic Stem Cells*. Amsterdam: Elsevier.

Latour, B. (1987) *Science in Action: How to Follow Scientists and Engineers through Society*. Cambridge: Harvard University Press.

Latour, B. (2004) *Politics of Nature*. Cambridge, Mass.: Harvard University Press.

Medical Research Council (2004) *Translating Research: Annual Review 2003/04*. London, MRC.

Michael, M., Wainwright, S.P., Williams, C., Farsides, B. and Cribb, A. (2007a) From core set to assemblage: on the dynamics of exclusion and inclusion in the failure to derive beta cells from embryonic stem cells, *Science Studies*, 20, 1, 5–25.

Michael, M., Wainwright, S.P. and Williams, C. (2007b) Temporality and prudence: on stem cells as 'Phronesic things', *Configurations*, 13, 373–94.

Mooney, C. (2005) *The Republican War on Science*. New York: Basic Books.

Moran, N. (2007) Public sector seeks to bridge 'valley of death', *Nature Biotechnology*, 25, 266.

Nowotny, H. (1994) *Time: the Modern and Postmodern Experience*. Cambridge: Polity.

Pickering, S.J., Minger, S., Braude, P.R. *et al*. (2005) Generation of a human embryonic stem cell line encoding the cystic fibrosis mutation deltaF508, using preimplantation genetic diagnosis, *Reproductive Biomedicine Online*, 10, 390–7.

Petryna, A. and Keinman, A. (2006) The pharmaceutical nexus. In Petryna, A., Lakoff, A. and Kleinman, A. (eds) *Global Pharmaceuticals: Ethics, Markets, Practices*. Durham: Duke University Press.

Potter, J. and Wetherell, M. (1987) *Discourse and Social Psychology*. London: Sage.

Rabinow, P. (1996a) *Essays on the Anthropology of Reason*. Princeton: Princeton University Press.

Rabinow, P. (1996b) *Making PCR: a Story of Biotechnology*. Chicago: Chicago University Press.

Scott, C.T. (2006) *Stem Cell Now: from the Experiment that Shook the World to the New Politics of Life*. New York: Pi Press.

Strauss, A.L. (1987) *Qualitative Analysis for Social Scientists*. Cambridge: Cambridge University Press.

Van Lente, H. (1993) *Promising Technology: The Dynamics of Expectations in Technological Developments*. Enschede: University of Twente Press.

Wainwright, S.P., Williams, C., Michael, M., Farsides, B. and Cribb, A. (2006a) From bench to bedside? Biomedical scientists' expectations of stem cell science as a future therapy for diabetes, *Social Science and Medicine*, 63, 2052–64.

Wainwright, S.P., Williams, C., Michael, M., Farsides, C. and Cribb, A. (2006b) Ethical boundary work in the embryonic stem cell laboratory, *Sociology of Health and Illness*, 28, 732–48.

Wainwright, S.P., Williams, C., Michael, M., Farsides, B. and Cribb, A. (2007) Remaking the body? Scientists' genetic discourses and practices as examples of changing expectations on embryonic stem cell therapy for diabetes, *New Genetics and Society*, 26, 251–68.

Wainwright, S.P., Williams, C. and Turner, B.S. (2006) Varieties of habitus and the embodiment of ballet, *Qualitative Research*, 6, 535–58.

Weber, R. (1990) *Basic Content Analysis*. London: Sage.

Williams, C., Kitzinger, J. and Henderson, L. (2003) Envisaging the embryo in stem cell research: discursive strategies and media reporting of the ethical debates, *Sociology of Health and Illness*, 25, 793–814.

Williams, C., Wainwright, S.P., Ehrich, K. and Michael, M. (2008) Human embryos as boundary objects? Some reflections on the biomedical worlds of embryonic stem cells and pre-implantation genetic diagnosis, *New Genetics and Society*, 27, 7–18.

Williams, S.J. (1995) Theorising class, health and lifestyles: can Bourdieu help us? *Sociology of Health and Illness*, 17, 577–604.

Zerhouni, E. (2003) The NIH roadmap, *Science*, 302, 63–72.

Index

Note: page references in *italics* refer to tables